Roberto Justus

Iatrogenic Effects of Orthodontic Treatment

Decision-Making in Prevention, Diagnosis, and Treatment

Springer

Roberto Justus
Department of Orthodontics
Universidad Intercontinental
Mexico, D.F.
Mexico

Conflict of Interest
The author declares that neither he nor any member of his family have a financial arrangement or affiliation with any corporate organization offering financial support or grant monies for this book nor does he have a financial interest in any commercial product(s) or services he discusses in this book (no conflict of interest whatsoever).

ISBN 978-3-319-18352-7 ISBN 978-3-319-18353-4 (eBook)
DOI 10.1007/978-3-319-18353-4

Library of Congress Control Number: 2015944187

Springer Cham Heidelberg New York Dordrecht London

Printed on acid-free paper

Springer International Publishing AG Switzerland is part of Springer Science+Business Media (www.springer.com)

This book is dedicated to my wife, Yolanda, and my children, Mauricio, Adrian and Tamara, for having made this work possible through their love and encouragement.

Preface

Orthodontic treatment success can be jeopardized by iatrogenic problems created during orthodontic treatment. The most frequent iatrogenic problem is white spot lesions followed by periodontal deterioration and external apical root resorption. This book addresses each of these three iatrogenic problems in individual chapters. Emphasis is given to the orthodontic treatment methods recommended to minimize or prevent these problems from occurring.

Mexico Roberto Justus

Acknowledgment

I am deeply indebted to Dr. David B. Wilkinson for his review of the manuscript, and to Dr. Ayax Martínez for his review of the clinical photographs.

Contents

Prevention of White Spot Lesions

1

Abstract

The most frequent iatrogenic problem in orthodontics is white spot lesions (WSLs). Maintenance of an adequate and constant presence of fluoride ions in the vicinity of the enamel on the periphery of bracket bases helps protect against the development of WSLs. Resin-modified glass ionomer cements (RMGICs) minimize the development of WSLs due to their continuous fluoride uptake from the environment and re-release, but the perception that orthodontic brackets bonded with RMGICs frequently fail due to low initial bracket shear bond strength persists. This perception is correct if the clinician were to bond these materials as recommended by the manufacturers, which includes conditioning the enamel with an extremely weak 10 % polyacrylic acid instead of the traditional 37 % phosphoric acid etch. In order to successfully use resin-modified glass ionomer cements, it is recommended to first deproteinize the enamel surface by applying 5.25 % sodium hypochlorite for 1 min to remove the acquired dental pellicle (which impedes proper etching of the enamel surface), followed by a 15–30-s etching with 37 % phosphoric acid (so the resulting etch patterns on the enamel surface are types 1 and 2, not type 3, thereby increasing bracket bond strength), and followed by moistening the enamel surface to further increase this strength. In following these recommendations, the clinician will minimize the risk to patients of developing lifelong WSLs and their consequences. In the final analysis the degree of damage provoked by WSLs is vastly more significant on the health of the enamel than the bonding and debonding process. It is the author's hope that this review of the scientific literature will help clinicians achieve the best results for their patients.

1.1 Introduction

Orthodontic treatment success can be jeopardized by the development of enamel white spot lesions (WSLs) on the periphery of, or beneath, orthodontic bracket bases. WSLs are clinically defined as opaque, white areas caused by the loss of

R. Justus, *Iatrogenic Effects of Orthodontic Treatment: Decision-Making in Prevention, Diagnosis, and Treatment*, DOI 10.1007/978-3-319-18353-4_1

minerals below the outermost enamel layer [1]. WSLs are the earliest sign of the caries process, which starts with enamel demineralization. The severity of WSLs can be classified numerically using a 4-point scale (Gorelick's scale) in which # 1 shows no enamel demineralization, # 2 slight, # 3 severe, and # 4 cavitation [2].

Brackets and bands create areas on the tooth surfaces which favor the increase of plaque and food accumulation due to the restrictive access for self-cleaning [3]. Carbohydrate fermentation by the bacteria in the dental plaque causes a decrease in the pH. This in turn results in the loss of mineral ions from the enamel to the oral environment, a process known as demineralization. Through the buffering action of saliva, the pH can increase again allowing the teeth to incorporate free ions. This process is called remineralization. There is a constant ionic exchange between the dental tissues and the environment, which will ultimately reach an ionic equilibrium. Progressive demineralization without adequate remineralization results in the development of WSLs [4, 5].

The formation of WSLs remains an unfortunately common complication during orthodontic treatment and is particularly prevalent in patients with poor oral hygiene. The initial lesions can be visible as soon as the 4th week after the placement of fixed orthodontic appliances [6]. Richter et al. [7] reported that nearly 75 % of patients who underwent comprehensive orthodontic treatment developed new WSLs because of prolonged plaque retention on the periphery of bracket bases. Therefore, the first step to prevent WSLs is to educate patients on the importance of maintaining proper oral hygiene throughout their orthodontic treatment. It is the orthodontist's responsibility to minimize the risk of patients developing enamel demineralizations as a consequence of orthodontic treatment. This can be achieved by brushing with fluoride-containing toothpaste after every meal and snack, rinsing daily with fluoride-containing mouthwash and by dietary modification, and limiting contact with sugar-containing products. Unfortunately, patient compliance is generally quite poor, particularly among the adolescent population.

The inhibitory effect of fluoride on bacterial activity and on demineralization of enamel has been well established [8]. The main mechanism by which fluoride works is by maintaining the plaque supersaturated with respect to fluorapatite, hence tipping the balance of the caries process against demineralization and in favor of remineralization [9]. Thus, continuous contact with fluorides is critical to protect the enamel against the development of WSLs during treatment with fixed orthodontic appliances. The presence of fluoride will minimize the ionic loss from the tooth structure until the pH of the plaque becomes as low as 4.5. At that level, even the presence of adequate fluoride concentration in the oral environment will have a minimal beneficial effect on the process of remineralization [10]. But before reaching such a critically low pH level, the availability of fluoride ions in the oral environment will enhance remineralization [11]. Resin-modified glass ionomer cements (RMGICs) can be used to bond orthodontic brackets. They have an anticariogenic effect because they release fluoride into the immediate environment of the bracket base, and they do so in a sustained fashion [12]. Therefore, maintaining an adequate and constant presence of fluoride ions in the vicinity of the enamel is critical to the ability of enamel to remineralize. It has been suggested that fluorides will have a substantial inhibitory effect on the rate of demineralization of enamel even if it is in the sub-ppm level, i.e., as low as 0.02–0.06 ppm [13].

The frequent application of fluorides is the most efficient method for preventing demineralization as well as enhancing remineralization of carious lesions. A potential method of providing a sustained concentration of fluoride ions over a prolonged period is to have a slow fluoride-releasing system incorporated in the bracket bonding material. Furthermore, the ability of some bonding materials for absorbing fluoride and then releasing it, acting as a fluoride pump, will help interrupt the development of WSLs, thus decreasing the risk of caries [14]. As a result, a few fluoride-releasing bonding systems have been developed. The fluoride ions released from these materials penetrate and diffuse into the tooth structure and prevent WSLs by reinforcing the mineral content of the tooth structure. The most effective fluoride-releasing materials in a descending order are glass ionomer cements (GICs), resin-modified glass ionomer cements (RMGICs), and compomers [14].

Resin composites to which fluoride has been added, called compomers, were not found to be effective in providing a sustained rate of fluoride ions [15, 16]. Thus, GICs were originally recommended as bracket adhesives to minimize, or even prevent, WSLs from developing due to their continuous fluoride release, but frequent bracket failure occurred due to their low initial shear bond strength (SBS). The reason for this low initial SBS is that glass ionomers harden through a slow acid-base setting reaction which requires 24 h to complete [17]. To increase the initial SBS of the GICs, 4–6 % photosensitive composite resin was added to be able to obtain a faster initial hardening of the adhesive's resinous portion through photocuring [18]. The addition of this resinous component converted GICs into RMGICs. These hybrid adhesives have allowed orthodontists to take advantage of the positive features of conventional GICs combining them with the mechanical and physical properties of resin composites.

Thus, the use of RMGICs to bond brackets is highly recommended because of their continuous fluoride uptake from the environment and re-release. However, these cements, in spite of the added resinous component, still have a relatively low initial bracket SBS [17].

To increase the initial bracket SBS to clinically reliable levels *when using RMGICs*, removal of organic material (deproteinization) from the enamel surface with 5.25 % sodium hypochlorite is highly recommended [19]. By applying 5.25 % sodium hypochlorite for 1 min, prior to phosphoric acid etching, temporary elimination of the acquired pellicle from the enamel surface occurs. This in turn allows the phosphoric acid to etch the enamel surface more effectively creating better etching patterns which increase bracket SBS [20–22].

The important topic of the acquired pellicle is presented later in this chapter. For the moment suffice to state that professional tooth cleaning by the use of a rubber cup or rotary brush with pumice does not completely remove the pellicle from the enamel surface; that the pellicle layer on the enamel surface confers resistance against chemical dissolution and attack by acidic agents, so 37 % phosphoric acid is not able to etch the enamel surface in areas covered with the organic material of the pellicle; and that temporary elimination (deproteinization) of the acquired pellicle from the enamel surface where the bracket base will be bonded is a must to be able to obtain etching patterns that allow effective bracket bonding with RMGICs.

To further increase bracket SBS, GC Corp., Tokyo, Japan, the manufacturer of Fuji Ortho LC, an RMGIC, recommends moistening the enamel surface with a water-moistened cotton roll before bonding, as verified by Rodríguez [23].

Clinicians typically require that a bonding material have sufficient initial bracket SBS to be able to tie arch wires into the brackets immediately after having bonded them, but since the glass ionomer fraction of RMGICs takes 24 h to set, clinicians prefer to continue using resin composites for bonding brackets to lower the risk of bracket bond failures, even if they do not provide a sustained fluoride release to protect the enamel from developing WSLs.

In the following subchapter, the reader will become aware of how severe and widespread the incidence and prevalence of WSLs are in individuals who had orthodontic treatment and will hopefully decide to incorporate the recommended modified method of RMGIC use to protect orthodontic patients against WSL development.

1.2 Detection

Among the most common methods of detection are clinical inspection and photographs. Quantitative light-induced fluorescence (QLF) has been recently suggested as a more accurate method of detecting WSLs [24]. The QLF method consists of illuminating the teeth with a blue laser light. Tooth dentin contains atoms called fluorophores which fluoresce green when illuminated with a blue laser light. This green light is blocked from exiting the enamel where a WSL is present. Thus, the WSL appears as a black area surrounded by green color. QLF technology is expensive so it is not widely used.

WSL detection can be a challenge when enamel decalcifications are in their initial stages. Before orthodontic treatment begins, the clinician should document the extent and severity of any WSL present through clinical inspection and with the aid of intraoral photographs. These photographs can be used for comparative purposes both during and at the end of treatment for patient education as well as for the documentation of their presence.

1.3 Incidence

A review of the literature indicates that there is a high incidence of WSLs that develop during comprehensive orthodontic treatment. Richter et al. [7], using the photographic method to detect WSLs, found that 72.9 % of 350 orthodontic patients treated with comprehensive orthodontics between 1997 and 2004 in the Department of Orthodontics at the University of Michigan had developed new WSLs. These 350 patients were selected at random from the photographic records of 2,300 patients treated at that institution. Boersma et al. [25], using the quantitative light-induced fluorescence method to detect WSLs, found that 97 % of patients who were evaluated immediately following comprehensive orthodontic treatment were affected with WSLs.

The next subchapter will address the question of WSL prevalence. It is an important subject because some reports indicate that a natural remineralization process occurs after orthodontic treatment which diminishes the prevalence of WSLs.

1.4 Prevalence

A review of the literature reveals that in spite of some WSL natural remineralization occurring post-orthodontic bracket removal, these lesions generally do not disappear. Van der Veen et al. [26] used the quantitative light-induced fluorescence method to determine whether WSLs diminish after orthodontic treatment (through the natural remineralization process). They found that 6 months after bracket debonding, while 33 % of WSLs did remineralize somewhat (lesion regression), the majority of WSLs remained unchanged, and 10 % worsened (lesion progression). Ogaard [27], in a study of 51 patients treated with comprehensive orthodontics, used clinical inspection to detect WSLs and found that the prevalence of WSLs on vestibular surfaces 5 years posttreatment was significantly higher than in a matched control sample of untreated individuals.

The results from the abovementioned studies indicate why methods of prevention or treatment for WSLs must be strongly considered.

1.5 Treatment

Methods to treat WSLs post-orthodontic treatment can be divided, according to Guzman et al. [28], into conservative and aggressive. The conservative treatment methods include oral hygiene instruction, dietary modification, chewing gum to increase salivary output (preferably gum containing xylitol, not sugar), remineralization with fluorides (in dentifrices, in varnishes, in sealants, and in mouth rinses with low-concentration solutions of less than 50 ppm), the use of antimicrobials (chlorhexidine), and casein derivatives (although recent research by Huang et al. [29] casts doubt regarding casein derivatives' effectiveness in remineralizing WSLs).

More aggressive treatment methods suggested by Guzman et al. [28] include external bleaching, micro-abrasion, composite restorations, and porcelain veneers.

Clinicians should recognize that the best policy is to prevent WSLs from occurring since the methods mentioned in the last paragraph are quite aggressive. It is therefore best to allow the natural remineralization process to take place as described in the next subchapter.

1.6 Natural Remineralization

Before attempting to use any of the WSL aggressive treatment methods, Guzman et al. [28] and Bishara and Ostby [30] recommended allowing the natural remineralization process to occur. Saliva contains minerals including calcium, phosphates, and fluoride ions, all of which help to remineralize WSLs [4, 5, 8–14]. During the potential natural remineralization period, good oral hygiene is essential. A reduction of exposure to sugared beverages should be implemented. Chewing sugarless gum is also recommended because it stimulates saliva production. In addition, daily oral rinses with low fluoride concentration and consumption of fluoridated water can be helpful. This should be combined with brushing teeth with low-concentration fluoride dentifrices to promote the remineralization process. Although it remains controversial whether high or low fluoride concentrations should be used, low fluoride concentration is generally recommended so that the external enamel surface remains permeable for the minerals in saliva to penetrate the damaged enamel surface [29].

It has been reported that 33 % of the WSLs improve with time as long as there are no enamel cavitations [26]. Unfortunately, many WSLs persist years after orthodontic treatment, in spite of the natural remineralization process [27]. Based on these facts, prevention or minimization of WSL development during the course of orthodontic treatment should be regarded as a factor of critical importance.

1.7 Prevention

Many methods have been proposed to prevent or minimize WSL development during orthodontic treatment. These can be divided into compliant and noncompliant methods [28].

1.7.1 Compliant Methods

Compliant methods include maintenance of good oral hygiene using fluoride-containing dentifrices, brushing well immediately after every meal and snack, diet modification to limit contact with sugar-containing products, and daily oral rinses containing fluorides. Continuous contact with fluoride is important because it protects the enamel by converting hydroxyapatite into fluorapatite crystals, which have a lower solubility in the oral environment than hydroxyapatite crystals [30].

In a systematic review published by Benson et al. [31], the researchers concluded that there is some evidence that the daily use of .05 % NaF mouth rinse, or bonding brackets with a glass ionomer cement, might reduce the occurrence and severity of WSLs during orthodontic treatment.

Topical application of stannous fluoride in particular may have a plaque-inhibiting effect by interfering with the adherence of plaque bacteria to the enamel surface. Tin atoms in stannous compounds also block the passage of sucrose into bacterial cells, thereby inhibiting acid production and diminishing the acidogenicity of plaque [32].

More recently, it has been suggested that the compound casein phosphopeptide-amorphous calcium phosphate (CPP-ACP) may also reduce the incidence of demineralization. The theoretical basis of this arose from the observation that dairy products are anticariogenic [33]. They work in a way similar to fluoride by maintaining the saturation of calcium and phosphate in plaque fluid, thereby discouraging the dissolution of these elements and also promoting remineralization if they are lost [34].

Unfortunately, compliant methods require patient cooperation, which is frequently lacking. Geiger et al. [35, 36] evaluated patient compliance in a preventive fluoride-rinse program. The degree of compliance with the home-care preventive protocol was poor in half of the patients, and less than 15 % of orthodontic patients used daily fluoride rinses as instructed.

1.7.2 Noncompliant Methods

1.7.2.1 RMGICs

In view of well-documented poor patient compliance, RMGICs have been proposed as bracket bonding materials due to their continuous fluoride-releasing properties throughout the orthodontic treatment.

RMGICs act as fluoride pumps due to the fact that they continuously absorb fluoride from the environment (e.g., fluoride in dentifrice, in oral rinse, and in potable fluoridated water) and subsequently re-release it precisely in the areas most susceptible to WSLs. These are the bracket perimeter and voids beneath the bracket base. In vivo [37, 38], ex vivo [39, 40], and in vitro [41] studies plus systematic reviews [31, 42] have documented that RMGICs do protect the enamel from the development of WSLs. These studies confirm that less demineralization occurs during fixed orthodontic appliance treatment with RMGICs than with traditional resin-based adhesives.

It is the author's opinion that orthodontic care should include protection of enamel from developing WSLs. This implies using fluoride-releasing RMGICs as bracket bonding agents. However, the current recommended method by the manufacturer needs to be modified to increase bracket SBS to clinically reliable levels. This can be achieved by *deproteinizing* the enamel surface with 5.25 % sodium hypochlorite (NaOCl) for 1 min, *etching* the enamel surface with a 15–30-s application of 37 % phosphoric acid, and *moistening* the enamel surface with a water-moistened cotton roll (the rationale for these three steps is explained in the following subchapters). Figures 1.1, 1.2, 1.3, 1.4, 1.5, and 1.6 show posttreatment intraoral photographs of patients who were treated by the author. These patients had bicuspid extractions followed by comprehensive orthodontic treatment using brackets cemented with Fuji Ortho LC, an RMGIC. It can be observed that no WSLs developed.

In addition to the use of fluoride-releasing RMGICs as bracket bonding materials, three other materials that also release fluorides include the application of fluoride-releasing varnish on the periphery of the bracket bases, the use of fluoride-releasing composite resin as a bracket bonding agent, and the use of fluoride-releasing sealants. These products can also be employed to help reduce the development of WSLs.

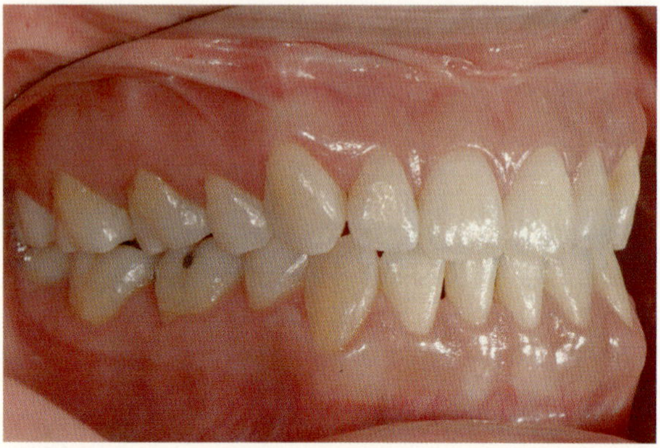

Fig. 1.1 Posttreatment intraoral right side view of a patient treated with extraction of four first bicuspids and full fixed orthodontic appliances for 24 months using Fuji Ortho LC as a bracket bonding agent. No WSLs can be observed

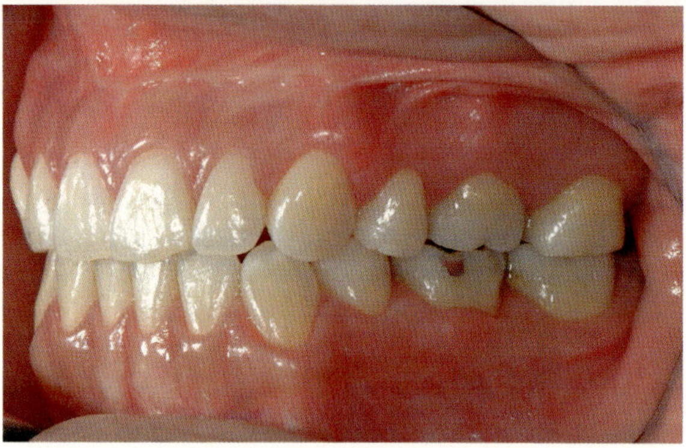

Fig. 1.2 Posttreatment intraoral left side view of the same patient

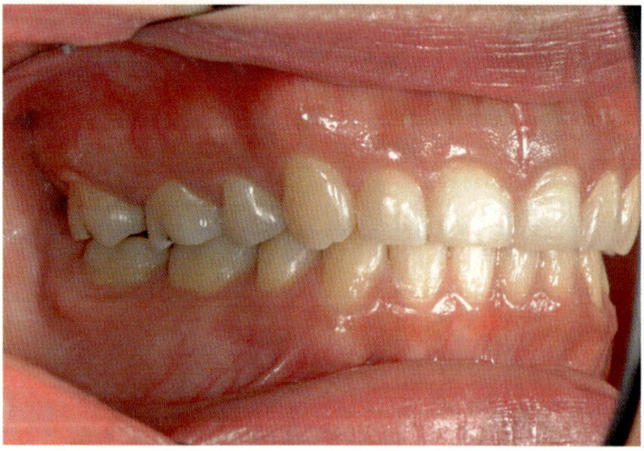

Fig. 1.3 Posttreatment intraoral right side view of a patient treated with extraction of four first bicuspids and full fixed orthodontic appliances for 28 months using Fuji Ortho LC as a bracket bonding agent. No WSLs can be observed

1.7.2.2 Fluoride-Releasing Varnishes

Schmit et al. [43] carried out an ex vivo study to evaluate the effect of a fluoride-releasing cavity varnish on inhibition of enamel demineralization adjacent to orthodontic brackets bonded with a composite resin (Transbond XT) and with an RMGIC (Fuji Ortho LC). Brackets were bonded to 48 extracted human third molars. Half

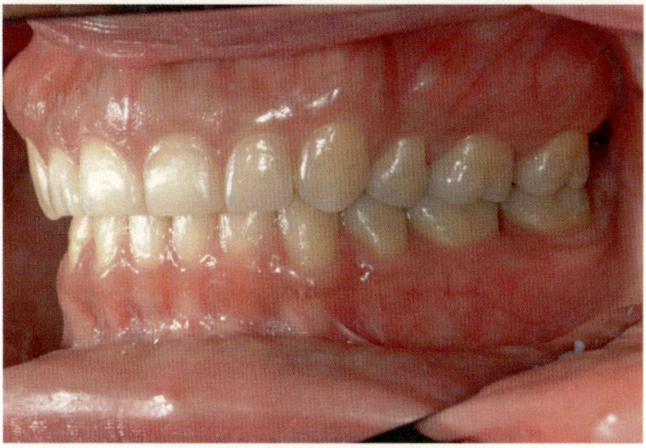

Fig. 1.4 Posttreatment intraoral left side view of the same patient

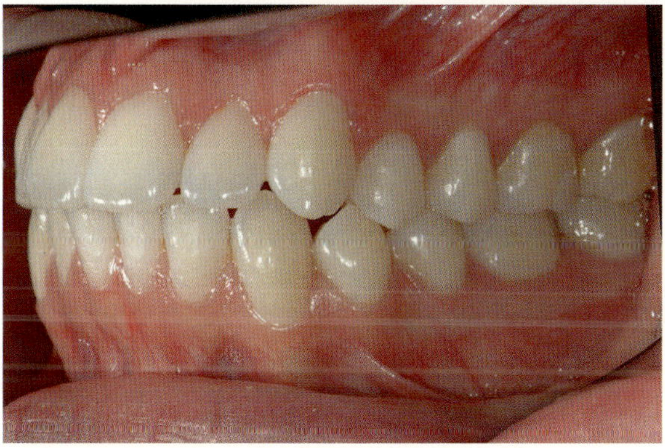

Fig. 1.5 Pre-treatment intraoral photograph of a patient who had previously been treated orthodontically using non-extraction therapy. The patient complained about having developed a double protrusion. In addition, the patient experienced three WSLs during this first treatment. These can be observed in the cervical third of the crowns of the second maxillary bicuspid and on the first and second maxillary molars

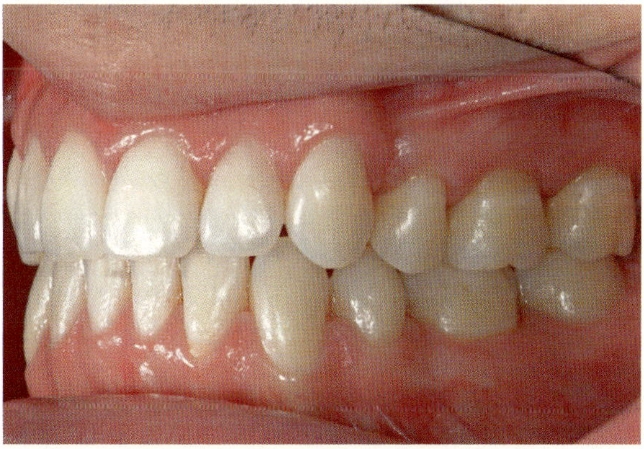

Fig. 1.6 Posttreatment intraoral photograph of the same patient after orthodontic re-treatment with extraction of four first bicuspids and full fixed orthodontic appliances for 30 months using Fuji Ortho LC as a bracket bonding agent. The same WSLs can be observed with no progression whatsoever and no new WSLs

were bonded with the composite resin and half with the RMGIC. Each group was further divided into 2, with half receiving an application of Duraflor (Pharmascience, Montreal, Quebec, Canada), a fluoride-releasing varnish. The samples were cycled in an artificial caries solution for an hour twice daily for 31 days. After each caries challenge, the teeth were brushed with a soft toothbrush to simulate normal mechanical wear of the varnish. The loss of fluoride varnish was timed. Teeth were sectioned longitudinally and photographed under polarized light microscopy. Mean lesion depth was measured. The authors reported that teeth bonded with composite resin showed a 35 % reduction in mean lesion depth when fluoride-releasing varnish was applied. Teeth bonded with Fuji Ortho LC showed no significant differences in lesion depth between varnish and non-varnish groups. Both RMGIC groups had 50 % smaller mean lesion depth when compared with the composite resin group without fluoride varnish. Samples bonded with RMGIC had lesion depths shallower near the bracket; depths increased as lesions extended farther from the bracket, illustrating a wedge effect—the protective effect to the enamel of the fluoride released from the RMGIC decreased with the increasing distance from the bracket. The protective effect of the fluoride released from the RMGIC decreased from the edge of the bracket out to 1 mm away from the bracket. The hypothesis that RMGIC, when used to cement orthodontic brackets to human enamel, can significantly reduce the depth of an enamel demineralization lesion adjacent to the bracket when compared with a composite resin-cemented bracket was supported in this study. The results suggest that RMGIC is more effective at inhibiting enamel demineralization around the bracket base than is the fluoride varnish. The varnish was removed from the teeth by brushing in just a few days; so it has to be frequently reapplied and it has a brown color that patients might find objectionable.

Thus, monthly application of fluoride-releasing varnishes is not necessary when RMGICs are used, but essential when composite resin adhesives are used, particularly in patients with inadequate oral hygiene. Guzman et al. [28] also suggested monthly application of fluoride-releasing varnish around brackets bonded with composite resins as a method to prevent WSLs in case of poor patient compliance with using preventive protocols at home.

Stecksén-Blicks et al. [44] carried out a clinical study whose aim was to evaluate the efficacy of topical fluoride varnish applications on WSL formation in adolescents during treatment with fixed orthodontic appliances, using brackets bonded with composite resin adhesive (Victory Twin APC II 3M Unitek, Monrovia, USA). The study design was a double-blinded randomized placebo-controlled trial with two parallel arms. The subjects were 273 consecutive orthodontic patients aged 12–15 years, who were randomly allocated to either the experimental or control groups with topical applications of either a fluoride varnish (Fluor Protector, Ivoclar Vivadent, Schaan, Liechtenstein) or a placebo varnish every 6th week during the treatment period. The outcome measures at debonding were incidence and progression of WSL on the upper incisors, cuspids, and premolars as scored from before and after digital photographs by two experienced and calibrated independent clinician judges. The sample attrition rate was 5 %. The mean number of varnish applications was 10 (range 4–20) in both groups. The incidence of WSLs during the treatment with fixed appliances was 7.4 % in the fluoride varnish compared to

25.3 % placebo group ($p<0.001$). The mean progression score was significantly lower in the fluoride varnish group than in the placebo group, 0.8±2.0 vs. 2.6±2.8 ($p<0.001$). The authors concluded that there were significantly fewer new WSLs in the patients that had the application of the fluoride varnish at each visit compared with the placebo varnish. The results strongly suggest that regular topical fluoride varnish applications during treatment with fixed appliances may reduce the development of WSLs adjacent to the bracket base and that application of fluoride varnish should be advocated as a routine measure in orthodontic practice.

Unfortunately, these frequent varnish applications demand extra time and work for both the orthodontist and the office staff and an increased cost to the patient, so the conclusion can be drawn that fluoride-releasing varnishes are not likely to be as efficiently used or as effective in protecting the enamel against WSLs as RMGICs.

1.7.2.3 Fluoride-Releasing Composite Resins

Composite resins with fluoride-releasing potential have been designed for bonding orthodontic attachments. They are called compomers or polyacid-modified composite resins [32]. Unfortunately, most of the fluoride from compomers is released and depleted during the first few days or weeks after bonding brackets. In addition, compomers do not have the critical ability to absorb fluoride ions from the environment [15, 16, 45–47]. Thus, fluoride-releasing composite resins do not provide the long-term cariostatic effect needed to prevent the development of WSLs.

In vitro data provided by Chin et al. [41] determined that RMGICs (Fuji Ortho LC and Ketac Cem μ) are more effective at inhibiting enamel demineralization adjacent to orthodontic brackets, because they maximized the release of fluoride and resulted in the least peri-bracket enamel demineralization in an artificial caries solution, when compared to a fluoride-releasing resin composite (Light Bond, Reliance Orthodontic Products, Itasca, IL).

Wilson and Donly [39] demonstrated that Fuji Ortho LC exhibits significant inhibition of demineralization adjacent to the bracket base, compared to Light Bond, a fluoride-releasing composite resin, and to Concise, a non-fluoride-releasing composite resin.

The conclusion can be therefore drawn that fluoride-releasing composite resins are not as effective in protecting the enamel against WSLs as RMGICs.

1.7.2.4 Fluoride-Releasing Sealants

Soliman et al. [48] measured the in vitro rate and amount of fluoride ions released from Pro Seal (Reliance Orthodontic Products Inc, Itasca, IL), a fluoride-releasing orthodontic sealant, over a period of 17 weeks. These researchers also measured the recharging ability of this sealant when fluoride ions were reintroduced into the environment. They found that this sealant did release fluoride ions. However, the release decreased significantly from a high of 0.07 ppm/week/mm^2 to a low of 0.01 by the end of the 17th week. They also found that this sealant had the ability to be recharged with fluoride ions from a foaming solution of acidulated phosphate fluoride, but not from brushing with fluoridated toothpaste. Unfortunately, the sealant had to be frequently recharged with the acidulated phosphate fluoride because even though the mean fluoride ion release was 0.354 ppm/week/mm during the 1st week after the fluoride application, it decreased to 0.014 by the 8th week.

1.7.2.5 Non-fluoride-Releasing Sealants

Non-fluoride-releasing sealants have also been developed. The application of these sealants around and/or beneath orthodontic brackets has been proposed as a method to prevent caries in orthodontic patients. Filled resin sealants have shown better retention and increased resistance to mechanical abrasion than unfilled resin sealants. Gizani [49] conducted a systematic review to evaluate the effectiveness of orthodontic sealants in preventing the occurrence of enamel demineralization in patients with fixed orthodontic appliances during treatment. The results were contradictory, with half of the studies showing significant reductions in the incidence of enamel demineralization for the sealed teeth compared with the control group, while the remaining half did not show any important differences. Gizani stated that it was impossible to make any reliable recommendations on the usage of these sealants during orthodontic treatment for the prevention of WSL development.

A recent prospective trial of 62 patients was carried out by O'Reilly et al. [50] to determine the effectiveness of a non-fluoride-releasing orthodontic sealant (BisCover LV, Bisco, Schaumberg, Ill) to prevent WSLs for the full duration of orthodontic treatment with fixed appliances. The researchers found a slightly lower incidence of WSLs on treated teeth (13.5 %) compared with the control teeth (17.7 %). WSL severity was nearly the same for treated and control teeth. They concluded that the sealant did not prevent all WSLs for the full duration of treatment but did demonstrate a clinically small but statistically significant ability to prevent WSLs.

The conclusion can be drawn that orthodontic sealants, whether fluoride-releasing or not, have limited and contradictory evidence to suggest protection of the enamel against WSLs and are not as well supported by the literature as are RMGICs.

1.8 Composition of Resin-Modified Glass Ionomer Cements

The main component of Fuji Ortho LC powder (LC stands for "Light Cured") is a finely ground fluoroaluminosilicate glass. The liquid contains polyacrylic acid, water, monomer, and an activator. The resin component of Fuji Ortho LC is a mixture of three monomers, with 2-hydroxyethyl-methacrylate (HEMA) being the major constituent. The HEMA provides for a sharp setting reaction of the material when exposed to visible light irradiation. In addition, a very small quantity of camphorquinone is contained in the liquid as a photoinitiator [51].

Among the advantages of RMGICs when used as bracket adhesives are the protection against the development of WSLs, the ability to bond in a humid environment (particularly useful when bonding brackets in the lower molar area), the ease of debonding brackets, the easier enamel cleanup since no primer is used, and the reduction of damage to the enamel surface during adhesive removal [51].

1.9 Setting Reaction of Fuji Ortho LC

The setting chemistry of Fuji Ortho LC, an RMGIC, differs from that of GICs, in that it involves both an acid-base reaction and a polymerization reaction. There are three stages involved in the setting reaction. The first stage is photopolymerization resulting from exposure to the light-curing unit (wavelength: 470 nm) which initiates free radical polymerization of HEMA, and two other monomers, to form a poly-HEMA matrix that hardens the material. This first stage, the formation of the poly-HEMA resin matrix, gives dimensional stability and an early set strength. The second stage reaction is a self-cure of the resin monomers. The third stage is the final setting of the acid-base reaction of the GIC fraction in the polymer matrix. The poly-HEMA and the polyacrylic metal salt ultimately form a homogeneous matrix that surrounds the glass particles. As a result the light-activated polymerization reaction is well harmonized with the acid-base reaction. Moisture contamination of the adhesive is encouraged in order to displace water-soluble monomers that may inhibit the glass ionomer set [52]. The light-initiated reaction also allows for early placement of arch wires, while the acid-base reaction occurs simultaneously, but far more slowly, and continues for a period of time after the mass has been cured by light irradiation.

1.10 Preparation of the Enamel Surface

Unfortunately, in spite of the addition of the photosensitive composite resin to the GICs, the initial SBS of RMGICs was still not high enough for clinical use. So it was suggested by Toledano et al. [53] that in order to increase the SBS, 37 % phosphoric acid be used for 15 s to etch the enamel surface instead of conditioning the enamel surface with the manufacturer-recommended 10 % polyacrylic acid for 20 s. These researchers found that brackets bonded with Fuji Ortho LC obtained similar SBS as composite resins 24 h after bonding, when the enamel surface was etched with 37 % phosphoric acid.

Ogaard et al. state that phosphoric acid applied to the enamel surface cleans the surface and dissolves the minerals to create multiple microporosities which result in micromechanical retentions; that it is important that the bonding material reach deeply into the etched areas and polymerize to give retention; that the bonding material must therefore be able to wet the surface, either by the surface having a higher tension than the bonding material or by using material that is sufficiently soluble in the components of the surface; and that phosphoric acid etching of the enamel creates this high surface tension that "sucks" the material into the roughened surfaces [32].

Thus, bonding brackets with RMGICs by etching the enamel surface with 37 % phosphoric acid, instead of conditioning it with polyacrylic acid, increases the bracket SBS during the critical 24-h setting time of the glass ionomer fraction in RMGICs so that the initial SBS is sufficient to withstand forces that otherwise would cause bracket failure.

Kakaboura and Vougiouklakis [54] have suggested that GICs do not adhere to the enamel through micromechanical retentions when conditioning the enamel with a 20-s, 10 % polyacrylic acid solution. They state that GICs bond chemically to the enamel through ionic bonding such as calcium bridges, hydrogen bonds, or van der Waals forces. These chemical bonds have a low initial SBS, however, which results in high initial bracket bond failure rates.

The recommendation by various researchers [19, 53] to etch the enamel surface, instead of conditioning it with 10 % polyacrylic acid, to create micromechanical retentions for adhesives, composite resins, and RMGICs, seems logical. However, despite phosphoric acid etching of the enamel surface, RMGICs still have a lower *initial* SBS than composite resins. Thus, clinicians have been reluctant to switch from using composite resin, an adhesive they have relied on since the beginning of their orthodontic education, to RMGICs. Historically, clinicians have tended to lay the blame for WSL development on poor patient compliance with oral hygiene instructions during orthodontic treatment and cited the risk of bracket failure rates as reason to defer the use of RMGICs, even though it is now known that RMGICs help minimize the development of WSLs. After review of the literature, the clinician should be more amenable to discontinue the use of composite resin in favor of RMGICs, as appropriate employment of RMGICs minimizes the risk of bracket bond failure while greatly reducing the risk of WSLs. Specifically, deproteinizing the enamel surface, etching of the enamel surface with phosphoric acid, and moistening of the enamel surface prior to bonding allow adequate SBS to minimize the risk of bracket bond failure to a clinically acceptable rate.

1.11 Increase in Bracket Shear Bond Strength with Deproteinization

Justus et al. [19] carried out an ex vivo study to determine whether deproteinization of the enamel surface, with 5.25 % sodium hypochlorite (NaOCl) before etching, increases bracket SBS of composite resin (Transbond XT) and RMGIC (Fuji Ortho LC). Brackets were bonded to 76 extracted premolars. Half were bonded with the composite resin and half with the RMGIC. Each group was randomized, with half receiving a 1-min application of NaOCl on the enamel surface. The findings indicated that by applying 5.25 % NaOCl for 1 min to the enamel surface with a microbrush (Figs. 1.7 and 1.8), followed by a 30-s acid etching with 37 % phosphoric acid and then moistening the enamel surface, the mean SBS of brackets bonded using Fuji Ortho LC was 9.64 ± 5.01 MPa, which exceeds the minimum mean tensile bond strength of 5.9 MPa, recommended by Reynolds [55]. In contrast, the Fuji Ortho LC group, in which NaOCl was not applied, had a much lower mean SBS (5.71 ± 3.87 MPa). Thus, if the clinician wishes to use RMGICs to prevent WSLs, it is recommended, based on the findings of this research, to deproteinize the enamel surface with 5.25 % NaOCl for 1 min before acid etching as there was a statistically significant difference between the 2 Fuji Ortho LC groups (control and

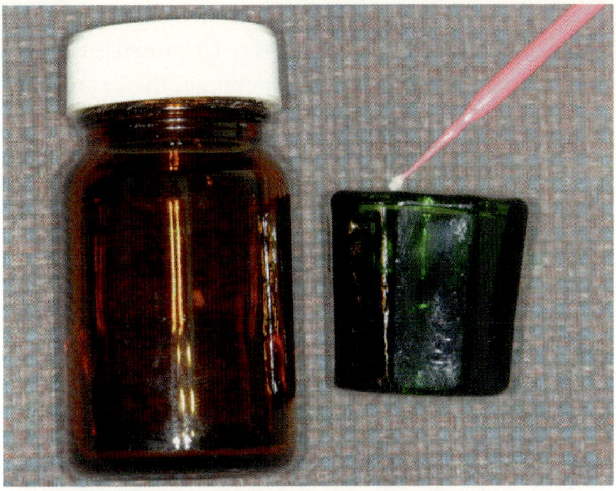

Fig. 1.7 Photograph on the left shows a glass container with a 5.25 % sodium hypochlorite (NaOCl) solution. This dark container helps prevent the deactivation of this solution by light. Photograph on the right shows a Dappen Dish containing the NaOCl solution and a microbrush used to transport it to the labial/buccal surfaces of the teeth

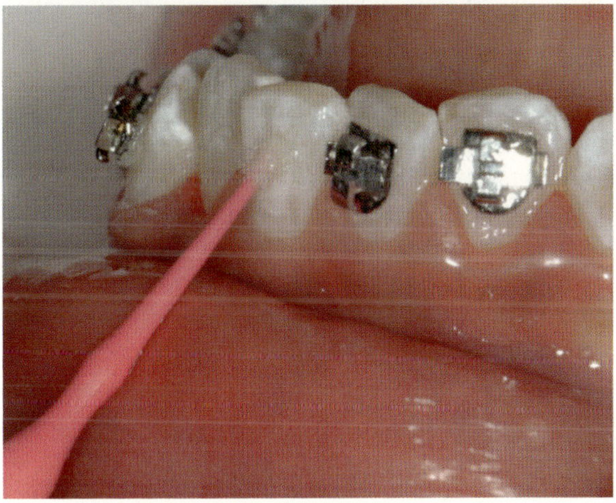

Fig. 1.8 Clinical example of enamel deproteinization by applying 5.25 % NaOCl solution to the enamel surface for 1 min with a microbrush. The objective is to eliminate the acquired pellicle so the 37 % acid etch can create improved etching patterns on the enamel surface to increase bracket SBS (Reprinted with permission from Justus et al. [19])

experimental). The mean SBS increased 3.9 MPa (from 5.7 to 9.6 MPa) in the Fuji Ortho LC experimental group (with NaOCl) while increasing only 1.3 MPa (from 8.1 to 9.4 MPa) in the Transbond XT experimental group (with NaOCl).

The authors believe that the small increase in the experimental Transbond XT group is because a primer is used in this system. The primer is an unfilled resin with a low viscosity. Even though the etching pattern is probably type 3 when no NaOCl is applied, the primer is able to penetrate deeply into the microporosities created during the acid-etching process on the enamel surface. This allows for the incorporation of resin "tags" into the enamel, thereby creating microscopic mechanical interlocks between the enamel and resin providing as a result adequate SBS, in spite of not deproteinizing the enamel surface. In contrast Fuji Ortho LC does not use a fluid primer.

Thus, if RMGICs are to be used, it is critical that the enamel etching pattern be of type 1 or 2 (to increase SBS), and not of type 3. The authors consider that the application of NaOCl to achieve a better etching pattern is important for RMGICs to be clinically useful. As the test specimens in the present study were stored in distilled water, the organic elements on the enamel surfaces might have been partially lost. Thus, the authors believe that the in vivo application of NaOCl might result in even greater SBS than demonstrated in this ex vivo study.

A modified adhesive remnant index (ARI) was used to quantify the amount of remaining adhesive. The scores for the Fuji Ortho LC group, in which the enamel surface was deproteinized, and the Transbond groups (with and without deproteinization) were similar. Bracket failure was seen more often at the bracket-adhesive interface, indicating a good bond between the adhesives and the enamel.

The ARI scores were of statistical significance and indicated that the brackets bonded using Fuji Ortho LC without NaOCl failed in a different mode than those bonded using the Transbond XT adhesive system and the Fuji Ortho LC with NaOCl. In general, bond failure for brackets bonded using Fuji Ortho LC without NaOCl occurred at the enamel-adhesive interface, whereas brackets bonded using NaOCl failed more often at the bracket-adhesive interface. Of critical importance, the ARI scores for the Fuji Ortho LC experimental group (with NaOCl application) and the Transbond XT experimental and control groups (with and without NaOCl application, respectively) were statistically indistinguishable, indicating an identical bracket SBS between composite resin and RMGIC bonded to an appropriately deproteinized enamel surface.

Bracket failure at each of the two interfaces has its own advantages and disadvantages. Bracket failure at the bracket-adhesive interface is advantageous as it indicates good adhesion to the enamel. However, considerable chair time is needed to remove the residual adhesive, with the added possibility of damaging the enamel surface during the cleaning process. In contrast, when brackets fail at the enamel-adhesive interface, less residual adhesive remains on the enamel, but then bracket failure probably occurs more often during treatment, disrupting chair time and prolonging the duration of orthodontic treatment.

The scanning electron microscope (SEM) results showed that the enamel surface, when first deproteinized with NaOCl and followed with phosphoric acid etching, was qualitatively rougher than when no NaOCl was used. Type 1 and 2 etching patterns (explained in the following subchapter) were observed on enamel surfaces of premolars deproteinized with NaOCl followed by acid etching (Fig. 1.9). Etching patterns of type 3 (also explained in the following subchapter) were observed in premolars where no NaOCl was used (Fig. 1.10). These results are similar to the ones reported by Espinosa et al. [20] in 2008. Enamel etching with 37 % phosphoric acid, after eliminating the organic elements from the enamel surface, probably allows more and longer adhesive tags to be created on the enamel surface. The additional and longer tags greatly increase the mechanical retention of adhesives to the enamel, particularly of RMGICs.

This study demonstrated that by deproteinizing the human enamel surface prior to 37 % phosphoric acid etching for 30 s and moistening the enamel surface after acid etching, the mean SBS of an RMGIC (Fuji Ortho LC) increased almost 70 % (from 5.7 to 9.6 MPa), 48 h post-bonding. This clinically important, and statistically

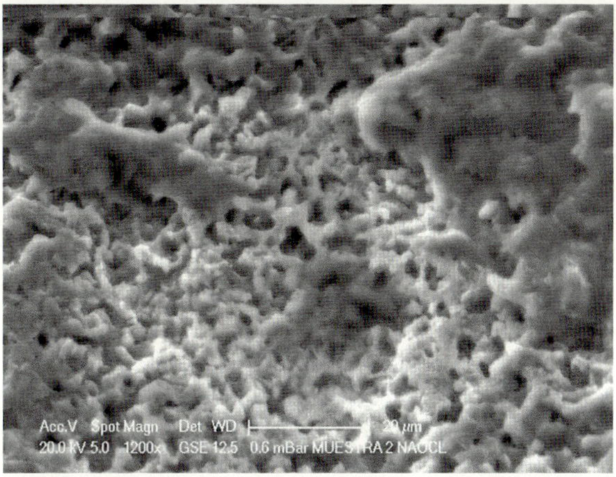

Fig. 1.9 1,200× SEM photograph of enamel moistened with 5.25 % NaOCl for 1 min and etched with 37 % phosphoric acid for 30 s. Observe type 1 and 2 etching patterns (Reprinted with permission from Justus et al. [19])

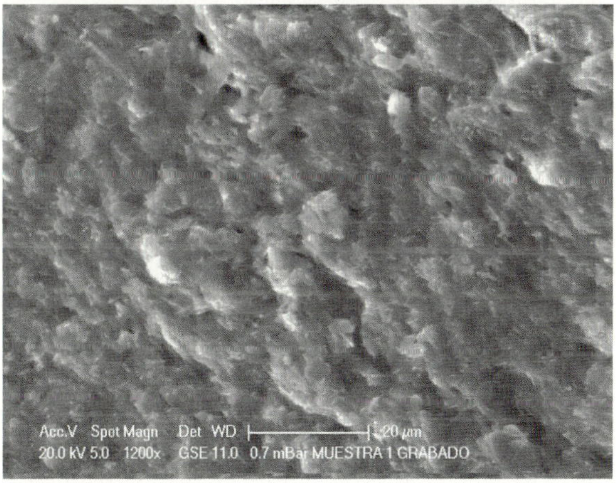

Fig. 1.10 1,200× SEM photograph of enamel etched with 37 % phosphoric acid for 30 s (no NaOCl was used). Observe type 3 etching pattern (Reprinted with permission from Justus et al. [19])

significant, increase in SBS finally allows orthodontists to reliably use RMGICs to bond brackets, thereby minimizing the risk of WSL development and also bracket bond failure.

To achieve successful bonding, *initial* bracket SBS is critical. This is increased if deproteinization, phosphoric acid etching, and moistening of the enamel surface are carried out before bonding brackets. A recent study by Vivanco [56] determined that the mean *initial* SBS, half an hour after bonding, was 9.85 ± 3.66 MPa in the Fuji Ortho LC group compared with 8.04 ± 3.13 MPa in the Transbond XT group, both groups with deproteinization of the enamel surface prior to phosphoric acid etching. This study further confirms the possibility of using RMGICs to minimize the risk of WSL development and put to rest the concern that orthodontists have of early bracket failure.

Enamel deproteinization is a prudent step in the overall bracket bonding procedure, whether RMGICs or resin composites are used. An improved marginal seal of the bracket base to the enamel is obtained with phosphoric acid etching to achieve type 1 and 2 acid-etching patterns, following deproteinization with NaOCl pre-application. WSL formation beneath and on the periphery of bracket bases can be minimized due to this improved seal.

1.12 Rationale for Deproteinizing the Enamel Surface

1.12.1 Enamel Etch-Pattern Types

Figure 1.11 shows a 2,000× scanning electron microscope (SEM) photograph of an enamel surface moistened with 5.25 % NaOCl for 1 min and etched with 35 % phosphoric acid, applied for 15 s. The high number of microporosities created in this good-quality etching pattern is characteristic of type 1 etching (in which the enamel rod, or prism, heads are dissolved). Figure 1.12 shows a 2,000× SEM photograph of an enamel surface moistened with 5.25 % NaOCl for 1 min and etched with 35 % phosphoric acid, applied for 15 s. The high number of microporosities created in this good-quality etching pattern is characteristic of type 2 etching (in which the enamel inter-prismatic substance is dissolved). These microporosities allow the adhesive to penetrate the enamel surface increasing the bond strength due to the many adhesive tags created. Figure 1.13 shows the 500× SEM image of an enamel surface etched with 35 % phosphoric acid applied for 15 s, without prior deproteinization. This low-quality etching pattern type, called type 3 (also known as *superficial etching*), in which some areas are well etched, many are not, or not etched at all. This type of inconsistent etching pattern offers little micromechanical retention resulting in an unreliable enamel surface for orthodontic bonding. Hobson et al. [22] reported that the majority of phosphoric acid enamel etchings carried out by dentists are type 3 etchings. These researchers demonstrated that the typical enamel surface etch pattern was as follows: 22 % of the surface not etched at all, 7 % with a tenuous etch, 69 % with type 3 etch, and only 2 % with type 1 and 2 etch. Ultimately, even though dentists pumice the teeth before etching, organic material (the acquired dental pellicle) still remains attached to the enamel surface, preventing adequate etching.

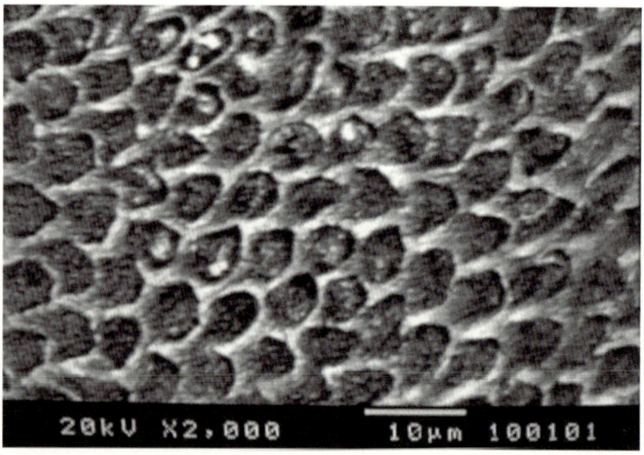

Fig. 1.11 2,000× SEM photograph of enamel moistened with 5.25 % NaOCl for 1 min and etched with 35 % phosphoric acid for 15 s. Observe type 1 etching pattern (Courtesy: Dr. R. Espinosa, Universidad de Guadalajara, Mexico)

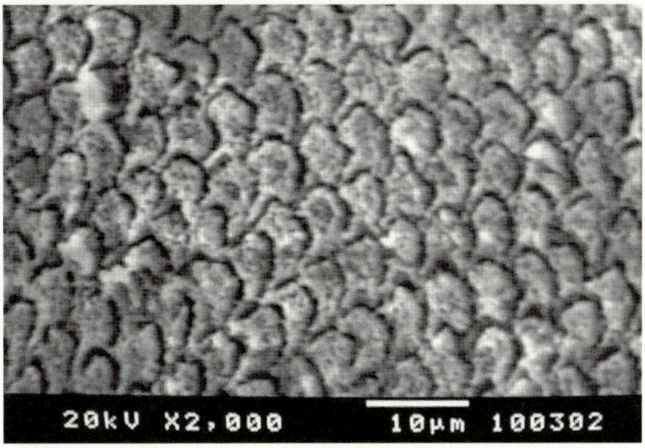

Fig. 1.12 2,000× SEM photograph of enamel moistened with 5.25 % NaOCl for 1 min and etched with 35 % phosphoric acid for 15 s. Observe type 2 etching pattern (Courtesy: Dr. R. Espinosa, Universidad de Guadalajara, Mexico)

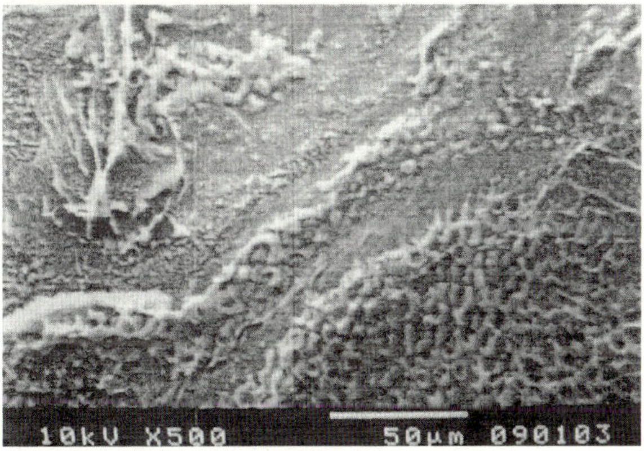

Fig. 1.13 500× SEM photograph of enamel etched with 35 % phosphoric acid for 15 s (no NaOCl was used). Observe type 3 etching pattern (Courtesy: Dr. R. Espinosa, Universidad de Guadalajara, Mexico)

The acquired pellicle derives from saliva and is the result of selective adsorption of salivary proteins and glycoproteins onto the tooth surface. In sheltered places it can be several microns thick but is thinnest on occlusal surfaces due to abrasion. The acquired pellicle is firmly attached to the tooth surface and is 1–3 μm deep. Although it can be removed by abrasion, this normally involves fairly extensive polishing. Professional tooth cleaning by the use of a rubber cup or rotary brush with pumice reduces matured pellicle to a great extent, but does not completely remove the pellicle from the enamel surface [57]. Basal pellicle layer has a higher resistance against abrasion compared to the outer pellicle layer. The full pellicle re-forms in approximately 2 h, once the tooth is back in contact with saliva. It penetrates the enamel forming the subsurface cuticle which is also 1–3 μm deep. The pellicle is permeable to fluoride ions and thus does not hinder fluoride uptake at the enamel surface [58]. The bacteria colonizing the teeth adhere to the pellicle rather than to the tooth mineral. The pellicle layer plays an important role in maintaining tooth integrity by controlling mineral dissolution dynamics at the enamel surface and confers resistance and stability against chemical dissolution and attack by acidic agents [59]. *Thus, phosphoric acid is not able to etch the enamel surface in areas covered with the organic material of the pellicle.*

Espinosa et al. [20] demonstrated that the percentage of type 1 and 2 etching patterns on the enamel surface increased from 47 to 94 % when organic material was removed from the enamel surface by deproteinizing human extracted molars with 5.25 % sodium hypochlorite (NaOCl). In order to achieve enamel surface deproteinization, these authors applied 5.25 % NaOCl to the enamel surface for 1 min, prior to phosphoric acid etching for 15 s. The resulting etched pattern area was 94 % types 1 and 2 compared with only 47 % without the use of NaOCl. Research was subsequently carried out by Justus et al. [19] (mentioned previously), which determined that deproteinization of the enamel surface with 5.25 % NaOCl does indeed result in a significant bracket SBS increase of 70 % when Fuji Ortho LC is used as an adhesive.

FDA-approved 5.25 % NaOCl for root canal disinfection and cleaning can be purchased at endodontic supply companies. Chemically similar NaOCl can also be obtained at supermarkets where 5.25 % NaOCl is commercially sold as a cleaning and bleaching agent worldwide. A popular brand name in North America is Clorox (The Clorox Co, Oakland, CA; pH=12.5). Examples of other brand names sold around the world are Candeggina (Italy), Domestos (Poland), 8+4 (China), Eau de Javel (Belgium), and Mistolin (Caribbean countries).

Endodontists have been safely using 5.25 % sodium hypochlorite *internally* to disinfect and clean root canals for over 100 years. Thus, orthodontists should have no reservations whatsoever about using this liquid *externally* on the enamel surface. It is advisable to apply this solution by rubbing the enamel surface, where the bracket will be placed, with a microbrush, taking care not spill the liquid on oral soft tissues. In the author's practice experience, even though the solution releases an unpleasant odor, the patient does not perceive this with the minute amounts used.

Another deproteinizing agent which has a similar action on the enamel surface as sodium hypochlorite is 10 % papain gel [60]. Papain is extracted from the latex of the Carica papaya fruit. The disadvantages of using papain gel as a deproteinzing agent are that it must be ordered through local compounding pharmacies and is usually more expensive than the NaOCl sold commercially.

1.12.2 Bracket Shear Bond Strength

Reynolds [55] determined that for a bracket adhesive to be clinically acceptable, it should have tensile bond strength of a minimum of 5.9 MPa.

Bishara et al. [17] carried out a study to compare the effects of time on the SBS of an RMGIC (Fuji Ortho LC) and a composite (Transbond XT) adhesive system specifically (1) within half an hour after bonding the bracket to the tooth and (2) at least 24 h from the time of bonding (when the adhesive has achieved most of its bond strength). Ninety-one freshly extracted human molars were collected. The teeth were cleaned and polished. The teeth were randomly separated into four groups. Group I, *RMGIC*, adhesive debonded within 30 min from initial bonding; Group II, *RMGIC*, adhesive debonded after 24-h immersion in deionized water at 37 °C; Group III, *composite*, adhesive debonded within 30 min from initial bonding; and Group IV, *composite*, adhesive debonded after 24-h immersion in deionized water at 37 °C. The results indicated that bracket SBSs were significantly greater in the 2 groups debonded after 24 h. This was true for both the RMGIC (mean = 8.8 ± 3.6 MPa) and the composite (mean = 10.4 ± 2.8 MPa) adhesives. On the other hand, the SBSs were significantly lower in the 2 groups debonded within 30 min of their initial bonding. The bond strength of the RMGIC adhesive (mean = 0.4 ± 1.0 MPa) was significantly lower than that for the composite (mean = 5.2 ± 2.9 MPa) adhesive. The findings indicated that the RMGIC adhesive had significantly lower initial bond strength but increased more than 20-fold within 24 h. In comparison, the composite adhesive had a significantly larger initial bond strength that doubled within 24 h. It is important to point out that in Groups I and II the enamel surface was etched for 30 s with 37 % phosphoric acid and in Groups III and IV the enamel surface was conditioned for 20 s with a 10 % polyacrylic acid solution.

In a follow-up study, Bishara et al. [61] found an increased enamel surface roughening when applying 20 % instead of 10 % polyacrylic acid, for 20 s, to condition the enamel surface. Their findings indicated that increasing the concentration of the enamel conditioner from 10 to 20 % significantly increased the bracket SBS of Fuji Ortho LC in the first half hour after bonding. The SBS increased from a mean of 0.4 ± 1.0 MPa to a mean of 3.3 ± 2.6 MPa, a more than 8-fold increase. However, the increase in the *initial* SBS was still not enough to be clinically useful.

It is important to point out that the term "conditioned enamel" means that the enamel surface has been cleaned and wetted with a weak acid (10 % polyacrylic acid) [61], while the term "etched enamel" means that the enamel surface has been undermined by a strong acid (37 % phosphoric acid) [32].

As mentioned previously, Vivanco [56] carried out a similar ex vivo study, using 90 premolars to determine whether enamel surface deproteinization prior to phosphoric acid etching and moistening would increase the SBS 30 min after light-curing brackets bonded with Fuji Ortho LC. This researcher determined that the mean *initial* SBS, half an hour after bonding, was 9.85 ± 3.66 MPa in the Fuji Ortho LC group compared with 8.04 ± 3.13 MPa in the Transbond XT group, both groups having been treated with deproteinization of the enamel surface prior to acid etching. This study confirms the adequacy of bracket SBS when employing RMGICs in this manner and should help allay the orthodontic concern of early bracket failure.

In spite of these new findings by Vivanco, in the author's practice a very light initial arch wire is employed since the acid-base reaction of RMGICs takes 24 h to set. This helps minimize the possibility of bracket failure during the first 24 h of the initial bonding when an RMGIC is used.

Composite resins have a relatively high initial SBS for several reasons. First, phosphoric acid etching creates micro-retentions on the enamel. Second, a primer is used which fills these micro-retentions creating tags (a mechanical interlocking between the adhesive and the enamel surface). Finally, the composite resin polymerizes soon after photo-curing providing sufficient early SBS to withstand both the occlusal and the orthodontic forces. The primer, a non-filled resin, has a low viscosity allowing it to easily penetrate deeply into the microporosities created by the phosphoric acid, forming resin tags which penetrate the enamel up to 20 μm, with most tags measuring between 10 and 20 μm [52]. These tags create the micromechanical retentions necessary for successful adhesive retention. They increase the SBS and thus minimize bracket failures. RMGICs, on the other hand, do not use a primer and, more importantly, use a manufacturer-recommended enamel conditioner, which is a very weak acid (10 % polyacrylic) that does not create micromechanical retentions. Ten percent polyacrylic acid only cleans the surface removing contaminants and debris and wets the substrate surface [62]. Kakaboura and Vougiouklakis [54] stated that RMGICs (employed without deproteinization and phosphoric acid etching) adhere to the enamel only through chemical bonds since the weak polyacrylic acid does not penetrate the enamel surface. The advantage of this more traditional method is that at the time of debonding no tags remain since no micromechanical retentions are created. The disadvantage is that the glass ionomer fraction takes 24 h to set, and during this time there is a higher probability of bracket failure.

In order to use RMGICs to protect the enamel from developing WSLs, it would be ideal for these adhesives to have tags for micromechanical retention. These can only form if phosphoric acid is used to etch the enamel surface. Fjeld and Ogaard [52] demonstrated that no visible tags are formed when RMGICs are cemented on enamel that has been conditioned with 10 % polyacrylic acid. Many studies have reported that etching the enamel surface with phosphoric acid, prior to bonding brackets with Fuji Ortho LC, resulted in bracket SBS that was within the range of estimated SBS values for successful clinical bonding [19, 53, 63–65]. Thus, it stands to reason that the more tags that are created and the longer they are, the higher the bracket SBS, particularly important during the first 24 h. While the presence of tags has not been conclusively proven with RMGICs, their presence would not be surprising with combined deproteinization, phosphoric acid etching, and moistening the enamel surface, prior to bonding with an RMGIC. The time course to full setting is also logical because 95 % of the material in RMGICs is glass ionomer [18], which takes 24 h to set since it hardens through an acid-base reaction.

For RMGICs to be successfully used as adhesives to bond orthodontic brackets, they require the creation of excellent enamel etching patterns, defined as types 1 and 2 [20]. Composite resins on the other hand are less dependent on the creation of as many microporosities because of the primer's ability to deeply penetrate the few existing microporosities associated with the type 3 etching pattern. By routinely deproteinizing the enamel surface to obtain an excellent etching pattern, regardless of whether a composite resin or an RMGIC is used, bracket failure rates will diminish.

1.13 Increase in SBS by Enamel Moistening Prior to Bonding with RMGICs

To further increase the SBS when using RMGICs, it is recommended to moisten the enamel surface after phosphoric acid etching using a water-moistened cotton roll or pellet. The reason for the increase in SBS when the enamel surface is moistened after acid etching is that RMGICs have hydrophilic properties. Moisture displaces water-soluble monomers that may inhibit the setting of the glass ionomer [66]. The manufacturer of Fuji Ortho LC also states that this RMGIC can be used successfully in a moistened environment. This was verified by Silverman et al. [51] in a clinical study in which the enamel was water moistened with a cotton roll.

The increase in bracket SBS by moistening before bonding with Fuji Ortho LC, as recommended by the manufacturer, was confirmed in an ex vivo study carried out by Rodríguez [23]. One hundred extracted human premolars were divided into 5 groups of 20 premolars each: Group I, *control*, using Transbond XT as the bracket adhesive and Groups II to V, *experimental*, using an RMGIC (Fuji Ortho LC) as the bracket adhesive. The characteristics of the 4 RMGIC experimental groups were as follows: Group II, without etching and without moistening, just conditioning the enamel surface with 10 % polyacrylic acid, as recommended by the manufacturer; Group III, enamel conditioned and moistened; Group IV, enamel etched with 37 % phosphoric acid but left unmoistened; and Group V, enamel surface etched and moistened. Twenty-four hours after bonding, the brackets were thermocycled and debonded using an Instron Testing Machine to measure the SBS. The average bracket SBS in the unetched groups (with and without moistening) had a clinically unacceptable low mean bracket SBS. The mean SBS in the unmoistened group was 7.84 ± 3.75 MPa, while the mean SBS in the moistened group was 7.92 ± 5.69 MPa. In contrast, the etched groups had clinically acceptable mean bracket SBSs. In the etched and unmoistened group, the mean SBS was 11.34 ± 3.63 MPa, while the mean bracket SBS in the etched and moistened group was 13.49 ± 7.61 MPa. The control group with Transbond XT had an average bracket SBS of 14.96 ± 6.71 MPa. The author concluded that Fuji Ortho LC has similar bracket SBS to Transbond XT 24 h after bonding, if the enamel surface is etched and moistened when using the RMGIC.

The fact that bracket SBS is increased by moistening the etched enamel surface [64] is yet another advantage of RMGICs because lower premolar and molar brackets are frequently bonded in a moist environment, since it is difficult to keep these areas completely dry.

RMGICs provide the advantages of sustained fluoride release and the ability to bond brackets in a moist environment (due to their hydrophilic properties). The latter advantage is particularly useful for bonding attachments to second molars. These molars are not being routinely banded, probably due to the difficulty and tissue impingement pain involved in banding. If these molars are bonded with resin composite, the bonds frequently fail due to saliva contamination of the enamel surface during the bonding procedure.

The American Board of Orthodontics has determined that many of the finishing problems in the clinical cases presented for certification arise in second molars [67]. By bonding attachments on second molars with RMGICs, the American Board of Orthodontics candidates improve their chances of approving the American Board of Orthodontics' clinical examination. Bonding second molars with RMGICs has a greater chance of success than bonding with resin composites because it has been documented [22, 50, 62] that the presence of humidity on the enamel surface, during the bonding procedure with RMGICs, increases bond strength.

1.14 Bracket Failure Rates

Many clinicians have reported high failure rates for brackets bonded with RMGICs. These failures have been mainly attributed to the low initial bracket SBS of RMGICs. Gaworski et al. [68] reported a clinical failure rate of 24.8 % for RMGICs. Hegarty and Macfarlane [18] in a clinical trial found four times higher bracket failure with RMGICs than with resin composite adhesive when brackets were in occlusion. The brackets with the RMGIC adhesive, however, were bonded using the traditional method, specifically without deproteinization, phosphoric acid etch, or moistening.

In contrast, some clinicians have reported clinical failure rates for RMGICs similar to the rates found with the use of composite resin adhesives [51]. Summers et al. [69] reported no significant differences in bracket failure rates between RMGICs and composite resin adhesives.

To the author's knowledge, no clinical research has yet been done on bracket failure rates when brackets are bonded with RMGICs, having the enamel surface been deproteinized/etched/moistened.

Investigators have evaluated various methods to increase bracket SBS of brackets cemented with RMGICs, such as using different enamel conditioners and concentrations, for different time periods, and increasing the light-curing time. Still, the resulting SBS was inadequate until researchers came up with deproteinization and etching of the enamel surface with phosphoric acid [19].

However, because the acid-base reaction of RMGICs takes 24 h to set, clinicians must abide by the following recommendations (guidelines) to be able to successfully use these adhesives, avoiding *early* bracket failure.

1.15 Clinical Recommendations for Bonding Brackets with Fuji Ortho LC (Guidelines)

To reduce the risk of WSL development during orthodontic treatment, it is recommended to bond orthodontic brackets with RMGICs. However, taking into account the fact that the acid-base reaction in Fuji Ortho LC takes 24 h to set, the following steps are recommended:

- Pumice prophylaxis with a rubber cup for 5 s per tooth.
- Rinse and dry.
- Apply with a microbrush 5.25 % NaOCl to two teeth at a time, rubbing the solution for 1 min on the enamel surface where the bracket will be placed (the saliva suction tip should be positioned in such a fashion as to suction away any NaOCl excess).
- Rinse and dry.
- Etch with 37 % phosphoric acid for 15–30 s.
- Rinse and dry.
- Wet the etched enamel surface with a moistened cotton roll.

- Mix powder and liquid as per manufacturer recommendations taking note that the operator has less than a minute or two (depending on room temperature and the ambient light) to position the brackets before the resinous fraction of this adhesive begins to harden/polymerize. It is therefore recommended to prepare adhesive for only two teeth at a time.
- Load the adhesive onto the bracket base and press it against the enamel surface *making sure that the bracket does not contact the opposing teeth while in occlusion.*
- Remove excess adhesive with a sharp scaler.
- Light cure and disc off excess adhesive.

Once all brackets have been bonded, tie in a very light wire (.010″ SS or a NiTi) avoiding full bracket engagement in severely malaligned teeth to prevent bracket failure, since the glass ionomer fraction of RMGICs takes 24 h to set. Keeping brackets away from occlusion is also critical to help avoid bracket failure. Hegarty and Macfarlane [18] in a clinical trial found four times higher bracket failure with RMGICs than with resin composite adhesive when brackets were in occlusion. The brackets with the RMGIC adhesive, however, were bonded using the traditional method, specifically without deproteinization, phosphoric acid etch, or moistening.

Brackets bonded with RMGICs using the traditional method have a much lower initial SBS than composite resins [17], so many additional micromechanical retentions must be created on the enamel surface in order to increase the initial bracket SBS and thus be able to successfully use these adhesives. To increase this inadequate initial SBS of the RMGICs, three steps have been recommended: deproteinizing the enamel surface with 5.25 % sodium hypochlorite, etching the enamel surface with 37 % phosphoric acid, and moistening the enamel surface, preferably with water since saliva contains proteins.

1.16 Ligation Methods in Relation to WSLs

Forsberg et al. [70] carried out a clinical study to determine whether the number of microorganisms in samples of dental plaque taken from the labial surface of maxillary lateral incisors was higher when the incisors were attached to the arch wire with an elastomeric ring compared with plaque taken from incisors ligated with steel wires. Twelve patients undergoing orthodontic treatment with fixed appliances took part in this study. A split mouth design was used; elastomeric rings were used for ligation on one side of the arch, whereas steel wires on the opposite side. The number of caries-producing microorganisms, specifically *Streptococcus mutans* and lactobacilli, in samples of plaque was recorded on five occasions during treatment and also once before treatment and once after treatment. The results showed that, in the majority of patients, the incisor which was attached to the arch wire with an elastomeric ring exhibited a significantly greater number of *Streptococcus mutans* and lactobacilli in the plaque than the incisor ligated with steel wire. The authors concluded that in orthodontic patients whose oral hygiene is not optimal, the use of elastomeric rings for ligation cannot be recommended, as they may significantly increase the microbial accumulation on tooth surfaces adjacent to the brackets, leading to a predisposition for the development of dental caries (WSLs) and gingivitis.

It is then understandable why WSLs occur so frequently, both due to the widespread use of elastomeric rings or chains to attach arch wires to brackets and to the use of composite resin bracket adhesives, which do not act as fluoride pumps.

1.17 Disadvantages of RMGICs

RMGICs have some disadvantages. Fuji Ortho LC requires a longer time to fully harden than composite resin (even though Vivanco [56] determined that the SBS was adequate 30 min after bonding), deproteinization of the enamel surfaces with NaOCl for 1 min (to increase SBS) is required, and mixing Fuji Ortho LC powder and liquid takes additional chair time (the manufacturer is now selling a no mix Fuji Ortho LC, which this author has not yet tried; it would be advisable to carry out laboratory studies before using it on patients).

Clinicians need to consider the properties of RMGICs to be able to use them successfully. Because of the recent improvements in the SBS with deproteinization and the fluoride-releasing capabilities of RMGICs, it is suggested that these adhesives should see greater use in bonding orthodontic brackets in the future. The advantages of using RMGICs far outweigh the abovementioned disadvantages.

1.18 Enamel Loss Associated with Orthodontic Fixed Appliances

A number of qualitative and quantitative studies of enamel loss during orthodontic treatment have been performed at each of the various stages of the bonding and debonding procedures, including at initial pumice prophylaxis, enamel etching, and cleanup after debond [71–73].

The purpose of pumice prophylaxis is to remove the organic enamel pellicle and any accumulated plaque before acid etching. The degree of enamel loss observed is typically on the order of 10.7 μm when prophylaxis is performed with a bristle brush in a slow-speed handpiece (10–15 s per tooth) but only 5 μm with a rubber cup [72]. Indeed, other work has supported the finding that enamel loss at this stage is determined more by the brush (enamel loss of 14.38 μm) versus the rubber cup (6.90 μm) than by the use of abrasive paste or slurry [73]. Whatever materials are used, in vivo studies have shown pumice prophylaxis to have no effect on bond failure rates with conventional acid etching and the use of a composite resin bonding agent [74] or polyacrylic acid conditioning and the use of an RMGIC [75]. Pumicing before etching is a controversial topic because many studies have concluded that it is unnecessary since the bracket SBS is not influenced. However, manufacturers recommend pumice prophylaxis before the use of a self-etching primer.

The magnitude of enamel loss during acid etching has been found to depend on the acid, its dissociation constant, the concentration, and the length of time it is in contact with the enamel surface [76]. Enamel surface composition and the presence of organic material (acquired pellicle) on the enamel surface also play an important role on the amount of enamel loss that an acid produces [20, 52]. The acid most commonly used is 37 % phosphoric acid, with an etch time of 15–30 s per tooth, in which case the enamel loss is typically in the region of 8.8–16.4 μm [77]. However, wide variations in enamel surface loss, from as little as 10 to 30 μm to as much as 170 μm, have been reported [78]. Self-etching primer on the other hand causes less damage to the enamel surface than the conventional 2-step etching and priming procedure because phosphoric acid is active for only 3 s in the self-etch priming procedure, being interrupted by the formation of a complex with the dissolved calcium [32]. Hosein et al. [71] determined that the median enamel loss by etching with the self-etching primer was only −0.27 μm, while −2.76 μm median enamel loss occurred with the conventional 2-step etching and priming.

Enamel loss can also occur during bracket debond and depends largely on the bracket material and method of debond used. There have been a number of reports of undesirable and alarming enamel fracture and loss at debond with the use of ceramic brackets [79, 80]. This risk is reduced with the use of metal brackets, but a small degree of enamel fracture (a tear-out) might still occur because of the micromechanical nature of the bond between a composite resin bonding agent and the acid-etched enamel surface. Therefore, some enamel loss will almost inevitably occur when the locus of bond failure appears macroscopically to be at the adhesive-enamel interface [81].

Enamel loss also occurs during removal of the residual adhesive from the enamel surface and polishing. Residual adhesive on the enamel surface after debond can be removed in a number of ways. If WSLs are present, Cochrane et al. [82] determined that less enamel damage occurs if they are remineralized before proceeding to debond. These researchers also found that the least damaging technique to remove the remaining adhesive on the enamel surface was with the use of aluminum oxide polishing discs since these remove the excess adhesive via abrasion rather than the gouging mechanism of fluted burs.

Hosein et al. [71], in an ex vivo study, measured the magnitude of enamel loss at each stage of the bonding and debonding process with the use of the conventional two-stage etching and priming process (in one group of 40 premolars with sound enamel) versus the use of the single-stage self-etching primer (in another group of 40 premolars with sound enamel). They reported that with pumicing and conventional etching, the cumulative median enamel loss was −2.76 μm, while with pumicing and self-etching primer, the cumulative median enamel loss was significantly lower, at −0.27 μm. At debond, there was a significant difference in the adhesive remnant index scores between the two groups, with more adhesive remaining on the enamel surface in the conventional-etch group. Enamel cleanup was carried out with one of four different methods: slow-speed tungsten carbide bur, high-speed tungsten carbide bur, ultrasonic scaler, and debanding pliers. It was during enamel cleanup that most surface loss occurred in both groups. However, there were statistically significant differences, with the greatest enamel loss in each case occurring after the use of conventional acid etching. The greatest median cumulative enamel loss was −14.3 μm, observed with the ultrasonic scaler after conventional acid etching of the enamel. Most enamel loss occurred with the use of the ultrasonic scaler or the high-speed tungsten carbide bur, and least was with the slow-speed tungsten carbide bur or the debanding pliers. What was not addressed in this study was the surface roughness of the enamel after each of the cleanup methods used. To achieve a similar surface smoothness as the untreated original, additional enamel would probably be lost in the polishing stage.

The conclusion can be drawn that self-etching primer causes less enamel loss of the enamel surface. Likely this is the result of three factors. Specifically, phosphoric acid is active for only 3 s, less adhesive remains on the enamel surface after debond, and less time is required for the removal of the adhesive. One has to keep in mind, however, that a non-fluoride-releasing resin composite is bonded over the primer, independent of whether it was bonded with the help of a conventional 2-step etching and priming or with the 1-step self-etching primer. Thus, greater risk for the development of WSLs exists with the use of a resin composite to bond brackets to enamel than with RMGICs.

1.19 Bracket Removal Recommendations (Guidelines)

At completion of fixed appliance therapy, one of the orthodontist's primary concerns is to return the enamel surface to as near its original state as possible [83]. The ideal would be minimal enamel loss at each stage of the process: pumicing, etching, debonding, and enamel cleanup, resulting in the enamel surface having the same degree of roughness or smoothness as the untreated original [82] with minimal discomfort and risk to the dental tissues.

Research has shown that the majority of damage to the enamel surface occurs during adhesive removal rather than during bracket debonding, pre-etch pumicing, and etching [71, 82]. The depth of damage to sound enamel, as a result of adhesive removal, has been reported to be as high as 150 μm [84] or even 170 μm [78]. If WSLs are present around or beneath the bracket base, enamel damage can be even more extensive [82].

Adhesive removal is easier when RMGICs are used because no primer is applied to the enamel surface. Therefore, fewer and shorter tags, if any, are created. If after enamel cleanup resin remnants (tags) are left on the enamel surface, these can discolor and produce an unesthetic appearance of labial enamel after debonding [52].

When self-etching primer is used in combination with composite resin, the tags created are shorter compared to those created with the conventional 2-step procedure (etching and priming) [52]. Although the etching pattern is claimed to be identical to conventional etching, the shorter application time (approximately 3 s) does not dissolve as much hard tissue or produce the same damage to the underlying enamel structures [32].

Of particular interest would be to determine the best way to remove the adhesive in the presence of WSLs because of the potential increased risk of further damage to the enamel. Surface enamel is lost at all of the four bracket bonding/debonding stages: pumicing (either with a rubber cup or a brush), etching, debonding (due to enamel tear-outs), and removing the adhesive, particularly in the presence of WSLs. WSLs debilitate the enamel so greater care is required to minimize the damage when removing brackets and the remaining adhesive.

Cochrane et al. [82] carried out an ex vivo study to determine the extent of damage to the enamel surface due to adhesive removal from sound, demineralized, and remineralized enamel, using four different removal techniques: aluminum oxide polishing disc, 16-fluted tungsten carbide bur in a slow-speed handpiece, 12-fluted tungsten carbide bur in a high-speed handpiece, and ultrasonic scaling. The adhesive used was self-etching primer (Transbond Plus) and composite resin (Transbond XT). WSLs were created by exposing the enamel on the periphery of the composite to an acidic solution for 12 days. Remineralization was carried out by exposing the demineralized enamel to a remineralizing solution containing 1 % casein phosphopeptide-amorphous calcium fluoride phosphate (CPP-ACFP) at 37 °C for 30 days, with the solution changed every 4 days. Damage to the enamel after the adhesive was removed with the four different composite removal techniques was assessed using white light profilometry, digital photography, and scanning electron microscopy. Transverse microradiographic analysis was used to determine the depth of the created WSLs, the extent of the demineralization, and the amount of mineral returned after remineralization. The results showed a 40 % increase in mineral content detected in the remineralized enamel exposed to CPP-ACFP as compared to the demineralized enamel. Sound enamel experienced the least amount of damage with the four removal techniques. Remineralization prior to adhesive removal significantly reduced the amount of damage produced by all techniques when compared with adhesive removal from demineralized enamel. As well, aluminum oxide discs were the least damaging to sound, demineralized, and remineralized enamel compared with all other removal techniques. They concluded that in the presence of demineralized enamel (WSLs), the use of aluminum oxide polishing discs was the least damaging method to remove the excess adhesive and that remineralization further reduced the amount of enamel damage.

Cochrane's recommended technique of removing composite resin from the enamel surface with an aluminum oxide polishing disc should also be applicable to the enamel cleanup of RMGICs, since by using deproteinization/etching/moistening the resulting bracket SBS is comparable to the SBS of brackets bonded with composite resin [19, 56].

Huang et al. [29] reported no difference in the improvement of the appearance of WSLs with MI Paste Plus (which contains CPP-ACFP), compared with normal home care. This result highlights the fact that minerals from saliva can remineralize WSLs as effectively as CPP-ACFP. It should be emphasized that MI Paste Plus was applied to the enamel of patients who exhibited WSLs after debonding. The patients had been selected for the study because they had WSLs. Thus, damage to the enamel surface during enamel cleanup might have been greater than would have occurred had the WSLs been remineralized before debonding.

Damage to the enamel surface is minimized by remineralization of WSLs prior to debonding. Cochrane's result of a 40 % increase in mineral content of demineralized enamel with the use of a CPP-ACFP prior to adhesive removal points to the importance of using a remineralizing agent to improve WSLs before debonding. This should reduce the risk of enamel tear-outs during debonding and also reduce iatrogenic damage during adhesive removal. It is important to point out that in Cochrane's study the damage to the enamel surface during the cleanup of remineralized enamel was approximately half of that produced by enamel cleanup of demineralized enamel. Remineralization might also be achieved using casein phosphopeptides to stabilize either amorphous calcium phosphate (CPP-ACP) or amorphous calcium fluoride phosphate (CPP-ACFP) because both increase the mineral content of demineralized enamel.

To remove the adhesive excess after the debond, Cochrane et al. recommend aluminum oxide polishing discs as the least damaging adhesive removal technique on sound, demineralized, and remineralized enamel. Aluminum oxide polishing discs compared favorably to slow-speed fluted tungsten carbide burs, high-speed fluted tungsten carbide burs, and ultrasonic cleaning. Aluminum oxide polishing discs remove adhesive via abrasion rather than the gouging mechanism of fluted burs. Cochrane et al. postulated that the less efficient the adhesive removal technique, the greater the likelihood of increased depth and area of damage, particularly when the remaining adhesive is surrounded by WSLs.

With conventional etching and priming, there is a higher potential risk for resin tags to remain on the enamel surface after debonding and cleanup, compared to self-etching primer and RMGICs. Resin remnants on surface enamel can discolor and produce unesthetic appearance of labial enamel after debonding [52].

Removal of residual RMGIC from the enamel surface is probably less damaging because this cement penetrates the enamel to a lesser extent than the adhesive (primer) used for composite resins, independent of whether the conventional 2-step etching and priming or the 1-step self-etching primer is used. This feature allows a safer debond, a diminished risk of enamel damage during adhesive removal, and a reduction of chair time.

It is noteworthy, although controversial, to point out that there are reports of no correlation between resin-tag length and the SBS of brackets bonded with composite resin independent of the method used for etching and priming the enamel surface [85–89].

It is the hope of the author of this book that this first chapter will create awareness among clinicians that they might diminish the incidence of WSLs by deproteinizing the enamel surface followed by etching with phosphoric acid and moistening the enamel surface in combination with a fluoride-releasing RMGIC.

Conclusions

- Significantly greater early bracket SBS can be obtained with Fuji Ortho LC as a bonding agent if the enamel surface is deproteinized (by applying 5.25 % NaOCl for 1 min), etched with 37 % phosphoric acid and moistened.

- When 5.25 % NaOCl is used to deproteinize the enamel surface, brackets bonded with Fuji Ortho LC have comparable early SBS to brackets bonded with Transbond XT.
- With 5.25 % NaOCl use, the ARI scores are similar when either Transbond XT or Fuji Ortho LC is used to bond brackets.
- Applying 5.25 % NaOCl to the enamel surface removes the acquired pellicle allowing the acid etchant to penetrate more effectively into the enamel, creating type 1 and 2 etch patterns. The increased SBS resulting from an improved etch pattern gives the orthodontist the possibility of using fluoride-releasing RMGICs as bonding adhesives to be able to protect enamel from developing WSLs, which is a major iatrogenic effect of orthodontic treatment. Protecting enamel health of patients by using the best available evidence should be an important goal of every clinician.

References

1. Murphy TC, Willmot DR, Rodd HD. Management of postorthodontic demineralized white spot lesions with microabrasion: a quantitative assessment. Am J Orthod Dentofacial Orthop. 2007;131:27–33.
2. Gorelick L, Geiger AM, Gwinnett AJ. Incidence of white spot formation after bonding and banding. Am J Orthod. 1982;81:93–8.
3. Chapman JA, Roberts WE, Eckert GJ, et al. Risk factors for incidence and severity of white spot lesions during treatment with fixed orthodontic appliances. Am J Orthod Dentofacial Orthop. 2010;138:188–94.
4. Samuel S, Rubinstein C. Microhardness of enamel restored with fluoride and non-fluoride releasing dental materials. Braz Dent J. 2001;12:35–8.
5. Serra MC, Cury JA. The in vitro effect of glass-ionomer cement restoration on enamel subjected to a demineralization and remineralization model. Quintessence Int. 1992;23:143–7.
6. Ogaard B, Rolla G, Arends J. Orthodontic appliances and enamel demineralization. Part 1. Lesion development. Am J Orthod Dentofacial Orthop. 1988;94:68–73.
7. Richter AE, Arruda AO, Peters MC, et al. Incidence of caries lesions among patients treated with comprehensive orthodontics. Am J Orthod Dentofacial Orthop. 2011;139:657–64.
8. Ericsson SY. Cariostatic mechanisms of fluorides, clinical observations. Caries Res. 1977;11 Suppl 1:2–41.
9. Hellwig E, Lennon AM. Systemic versus topical fluoride. Caries Res. 2004;38:258–62.
10. Ogaard B, Rolla G. Cariological aspects of treatment with fixed orthodontic appliances. 2. New concepts on cariostatic mechanisms of topical fluoride. Kieferorthopaedische Mitt. 1993;6:45–51.
11. Vieira AR, Souza PR, Modesto A. Fluoride uptake and release by composites and glass ionomers in a high caries challenge situation. Am J Dent. 1999;12:14–8.
12. Dionysopoulos P, Kotsanos N, Pataridou A. Fluoride release and uptake by four new fluoride releasing restorative materials. J Oral Rehabil. 2003;30:866–71.
13. Ten Cate JM. Current concepts on the theories of the mechanism of action of fluoride. Acta Odontol Scand. 1999;57:325–9.
14. Creanor SL, Carruthers LMC, Sauders WP, et al. Fluoride uptake and release characteristics of glass ionomer cements. Caries Res. 1994;28:322–8.
15. Dionysopoulos P, Kotsanos N, Koubia E, et al. Inhibition of demineralization in vitro around fluoride releasing materials. J Oral Rehabil. 2003;30:1216–21.

16. Miranda L, Weidlich P, Samuel S, et al. Fluoride release from restorative materials coated with an adhesive. Braz Dent J. 2002;13:39–43.
17. Bishara SE, VonWald L, Olsen ME, et al. Effect of time on the shear bond strength of glass ionomer and composite orthodontic adhesives. Am J Orthod Dentofacial Orthop. 1999;116:616–20.
18. Hegarty DJ, Macfarlane TV. In vivo bracket retention comparison of a resin-modified bracket adhesive system after a year. Am J Orthod Dentofacial Orthop. 2002;121:496–501.
19. Justus R, Cubero T, Ondarza R, et al. A new technique with sodium hypochlorite to increase bracket shear bond strength of fluoride-releasing resin-modified glass ionomer cements: comparing shear bond strength of two adhesive systems with enamel surface deproteinization before etching. Semin Orthod. 2010;16:66–75.
20. Espinosa R, Valencia R, Uribe M. Enamel deproteinization and its effect on acid etching. An in vitro study. J Clin Pediatr Dent. 2008;33:13–20.
21. Silverstone LM, Saxton CA, Dogon IL, et al. Variation in the pattern of acid etching of human dental enamel examined by scanning electron microscopy. Caries Res. 1975;9:373–87.
22. Hobson RS, Rugg-Gunn AJ, Booth TA. Acid etch patterns on the buccal surface of human permanent teeth. Arch Oral Biol. 2002;47:407–12.
23. Rodríguez J. Bond strength of a glass ionomer cement and a light cured composite: an *ex vivo* study. MS Thesis, Intercontinental University, Mexico City; 1997.
24. Al-Khateeb S, Forsberg CM, de Jong EJ, et al. A longitudinal laser fluorescence study of white spot lesions in orthodontic patients. Am J Orthod Dentofacial Orthop. 1998;113:595–602.
25. Boersma JG, van der Veen MH, Lagerweij MD, et al. Caries prevalence measured with quantitative light-induced fluorescence after treatment with fixed orthodontic appliances: influencing factors. Caries Res. 2005;39:41–7.
26. van der Veen MH, Mattousch T, Boersma JG. Longitudinal development of caries lesions after orthodontic treatment evaluated by quantitative light-induced fluorescence. Am J Orthod Dentofacial Orthop. 2007;131:223–8.
27. Ogaard B. Prevalence of white spot lesions in 19-year olds: a study on untreated and orthodontically treated persons 5 years after treatment. Am J Orthod Dentofacial Orthop. 1989;96:423–7.
28. Guzman-Armstrong S, Chalmers J, Warren JJ. Readers' forum, ask us. Am J Orthod Dentofacial Orthop. 2010;138:690–6.
29. Huang GJ, Roloff-Chiang B, Mills BE, et al. Effectiveness of MI Paste Plus and PreviDent fluoride varnish for treatment of white spot lesions: a randomized controlled trial. Am J Orthod Dentofacial Orthop. 2013;143:31–41.
30. Bishara SE, Ostby AW. White spot lesions: formation, prevention and treatment. Semin Orthod. 2008;14:174–82.
31. Benson PE, Shah AA, Millett DT, et al. Fluorides, orthodontics and demineralization: a systematic review. J Orthod. 2005;32:102–14.
32. Ogaard B, Bishara SE, Duschner H. Enamel effects during bonding-debonding and treatment with fixed appliances. In: Graber TM, Eliades T, Athanasiou A, editors. Risk management in orthodontics: experts guide to malpractice. Chicago: Quintessence Publishing Co, Inc.; 2004. p. 19–46.
33. Benson PE. Prevention of demineralization during orthodontic treatment with fluoride-containing materials or casein phosphopeptide-amorphous calcium phosphate. In: Huang GJ, Richmond S, Vig KWL, editors. Evidence-based orthodontics. Chichester: Wiley-Blackwell Publishing Ltd.; 2011. p. 149–65.
34. Reynolds EC. Remineralization of enamel subsurface lesions by casein phosphopeptide-stabilized calcium phosphate solutions. J Dent Res. 1997;76:1587–95.
35. Geiger AM, Gorelick L, Gwinnet AJ, et al. The effect of a fluoride program on white spot formation during orthodontic treatment. Am J Orthod Dentofacial Orthop. 1988;93:29–37.
36. Geiger AM, Gorelick L, Gwinnet AJ, et al. Reducing white spot lesions in orthodontic populations with fluoride rinsing. Am J Orthod Dentofacial Orthop. 1992;101:403–7.
37. Marcusson A, Norevall LI, Persson M. White spot reduction when using a glass ionomer cement for bonding in orthodontics: a longitudinal and comparative study. Eur J Orthod. 1997;19:233–42.

38. Czochrowska EM, Ogaard B, Duschner H, et al. Cariostatic effect of a light-cured, resin-reinforced glass-ionomer for bonding orthodontic brackets in vivo. A combined study using microradiography and confocal laser scanning microscopy. J Orofac Orthop. 1998;59:265–73.
39. Wilson RM, Donly KJ. Demineralization around orthodontic brackets bonded with resin-modified glass ionomer cement and fluoride-releasing resin composite. J Pediatr Dent. 2001;23:255–9.
40. Sudjalim TR, Woods MG, Manton DJ, et al. Prevention of demineralization around orthodontic brackets in vitro. Am J Orthod Dentofacial Orthop. 2007;131:705.e1–9.
41. Chin MYH, Sandham A, Rumachik EN, et al. Fluoride release and cariostatic potential of orthodontic adhesives with and without daily fluoride rinsing. Am J Orthod Dentofacial Orthop. 2009;136:547–53.
42. Rogers S, Chadwick B, Treasure E. Fluoride-containing orthodontic adhesives and decalcification in patients with fixed appliances: a systematic review. Am J Orthod Dentofacial Orthop. 2010;138:390.e1–8.
43. Schmit JL, Staley RN, Wefel JS, et al. Effect of fluoride varnish on demineralization adjacent to orthodontic brackets. Am J Orthod Dentofacial Orthop. 1999;116:159–67.
44. Stecksén-Blicks C, Renfors G, Oscarson ND, et al. Caries-preventive effectiveness of a fluoride varnish: a randomized controlled trial in adolescents with fixed orthodontic appliances. Caries Res. 2007;41:455–9.
45. Buyukyilmaz T, Ogaard B. Caries-preventive effects of fluoride-releasing materials. Adv Dent Res. 1995;9:377–83.
46. Steckel SE, Rueggeberg FA, Whitford GM. Effect of cure mode and fluoride content on bracket debonding. Angle Orthod. 1999;69:282–7.
47. Vorhies BA, Donly KJ, Staley RN, et al. Enamel demineralization adjacent to orthodontic brackets bonded with hybrid glass ionomer cements: an in vitro study. Am J Orthod Dentofacial Orthop. 1998;114:668–74.
48. Soliman MM, Bishara SE, Wefel J. Fluoride release rate from an orthodontic sealant and its clinical implications. Angle Orthod. 2006;76:282–8.
49. Gizani R. The effect of sealant on prevention of enamel demineralization in patients with fixed orthodontic appliances: a systematic review. South Eur J Orthod Dentofac Res. 2014;1:3–9.
50. O'Reilly MT, De Jesús J, Hatch JP. Effectiveness of a sealant compared with no sealant in preventing enamel demineralization in patients with fixed orthodontic appliances: a prospective clinical trial. Am J Orthod Dentofacial Orthop. 2013;143:837–44.
51. Silverman E, Cohen M, Demke R, et al. A new light-cured glass ionomer cement that bonds brackets to teeth without etching in the presence of saliva. Am J Orthod Dentofacial Orthop. 1995;108:231–6.
52. Fjeld M, Ogaard B. Scanning electron microscopic evaluation of enamel surfaces exposed to 3 orthodontic bonding systems. Am J Orthod Dentofacial Orthop. 2006;130:575–81.
53. Toledano M, Osorio R, Osorio E, et al. Bond strength of orthodontic brackets using different light and self-curing cements. Angle Orthod. 2003;73:56–63.
54. Kakaboura A, Vougiouklakis G. Cements in orthodontics. In: Brantley WA, Eliades T, editors. Orthodontic materials. Stuttgart: Thieme; 2001. p. 221–40.
55. Reynolds IR. A review of direct orthodontic bonding. Br J Orthod. 1979;2:171–8.
56. Vivanco C. Effect of time on the shear bond strength of an ionomer and a composite: an ex-vivo study. MS Thesis, Intercontinental University, Mexico City; 2014.
57. Hannig M, Bösmann K. Die Abrasivität des Pellikels unter klinischen Gesichtspunkten. Dtsch Zahnarztl Z. 1987;42:1015–20.
58. Cruz R, Rolla G. Deposition of alkali-soluble fluoride on enamel surface with or without pellicle. Scand J Dent Res. 1991;99:96–9.
59. Hannig M, Joiner A. The structure, function and properties of the acquired pellicle. In: Duckworth RM, editor. The teeth and their environment, Monographs in oral science, vol. 19. Basel: Karger; 2006. p. 29–64.
60. Pithon M, Ferraz CS, de Oliveira GC. Effect of 10 % papain gel on enamel deproteinization before the bonding procedure. Angle Orthod. 2012;82:541–5.

61. Bishara SE, von Wald L, Laffoon JF, et al. Effect of changing enamel conditioner concentration on the shear bond strength of a resin-modified glass ionomer adhesive. Am J Orthod Dentofacial Orthop. 2000;118:311–6.
62. Powis DR, Folleras T, Merson SA, et al. Improved adhesion of a glass ionomer cement to dentin and enamel. J Dent Res. 1982;61:1416–22.
63. Flores AR, Saez EG, Barcelo F. Metallic bracket to enamel bonding with a photopolymerizable resin-reinforced glass ionomer. Am J Orthod Dentofacial Orthop. 1999;116:514–7.
64. Larmour CJ, Stirrups DR. An Ex vivo assessment of a Resin-modified Glass Ionomer Cement in Relation to Bonding Technique. J Orthod. 2001;28:207–10.
65. Godoy-Becerra J, Vieira S, Gonzaga Oliveira JH, et al. Shear Bond Strength of Resin-modified Glass Ionomer Cement with Saliva Present and Different Enamel Pretreatments. Angle Orthod. 2006;76:470–4.
66. Cacciafesta V, Jost-Brinkman PG, Sussenberger U, et al. Effects of saliva and water contamination on the enamel shear bond strength of a light-cured glass ionomer cement. Am J Orthod Dentofacial Orthop. 1998;113:402–7.
67. Casko JS, Vaden JL, Kokich VG, et al. Objective grading system for dental casts and panoramic radiographs. Am J Orthod Dentofacial Orthop. 1998;114:589–99.
68. Gaworski M, Weinstein M, Borislow A, et al. Decalcification and bond failure: a comparison of a glass ionomer and a composite resin bonding system in vivo. Am J Orthod Dentofacial Orthop. 1999;116:518–21.
69. Summers A, Kao E, Gilmore J, Gunel E, Ngan P. Comparison of bond strength between a conventional resin adhesive and a resin-modified glass ionomer adhesive: an in vitro and in vivo study. Am J Orthod Dentofacial Orthop. 2004;126:200–6.
70. Forsberg CM, Brattström V, Malmberg E, et al. Ligature wires and elastomeric rings: two methods of ligation, and their association with microbial colonization of Streptococcus mutans and Lactobacilli. Eur J Orthod. 1991;13:416–20.
71. Hosein I, Sherriff M, Ireland AJ. Enamel loss during bonding, debonding, and clean-up with use of a self-etching primer. Am J Orthod Dentofacial Orthop. 2004;126:717–24.
72. Pus MD, Way DC. Enamel loss due to orthodontic bonding with filled and unfilled resins using various clean-up techniques. Am J Orthod. 1980;77:269–83.
73. Thompson RE, Way DC. Enamel loss due to prophylaxis and multiple bonding/debonding of orthodontic brackets. Am J Orthod. 1981;79:282–95.
74. Barry GRP. A clinical investigation of the effects of omission of pumice prophylaxis on band and bond failure. Br J Orthod. 1995;22:245–8.
75. Ireland AJ, Sherriff M. The effect of pumicing on the in vivo use of a resin modified glass poly (alkenoate) cement and a conventional no-mix composite for bonding orthodontic brackets. J Orthod. 2002;29:217–20.
76. Uno S, Finger WJ. Effect of acid etchant composition and etch duration on enamel loss and resin composite bonding. Am J Orthod. 1995;8:165–9.
77. Legler LR, Retief DH, Bradley EL, et al. Effects of phosphoric acid concentration and etch duration on enamel depth of etch: an in vitro study. Am J Orthod Dentofacial Orthop. 1990;98:154–60.
78. Diedrich P. Enamel alterations from bracket bonding and debonding: a study with the scanning electron microscope. Am J Orthod. 1981;79:500–23.
79. Joseph VP, Rossouw PE. The shear bond strengths of stainless steel orthodontic brackets bonded to teeth with orthodontic composite resin and various fissure sealants. Am J Orthod Dentofacial Orthop. 1990;98:66–71.
80. Jeroudi MT. Enamel fracture caused by ceramic brackets. Am J Orthod Dentofacial Orthop. 1991;99:97–9.
81. Redd TB, Shivapuja PK. Debonding ceramic brackets: effects on enamel. J Clin Orthod. 1991;25:475–81.
82. Cochrane N, Ratneser S, Reynolds EC. Effect of different orthodontic adhesive removal techniques on sound, demineralized and remineralized enamel. Aust Dent J. 2012;57:365–72.
83. Campbell PM. Enamel surface after orthodontic bracket debonding. Angle Orthod. 1995;2:103–10.

84. Krell KV, Courey JM, Bishara SE. Orthodontic bracket removal using conventional and ultrasonic debonding techniques, enamel loss, and time requirements. Am J Orthod. 1993;103: 258–66.
85. Torii Y, Hikasa R, Iwata S, et al. Enamel tensile bond strength and morphology of resin-enamel interface created by acid etching system with or without moisture and self-etching priming system. J Oral Rehabil. 2002;29:528–33.
86. Mattick CR, Hobson RS. A comparative micro-topographic study of the buccal enamel of different tooth types. J Orthod. 2000;27:143–8.
87. Barkmeier WW, Gwinnett AJ, Shaffer SE. Effects of reduced acid concentration and etching time on bond strength and enamel morphology. J Clin Orthod. 1987;21:395–8.
88. Legler LR, Retief DH, Bradley EL, et al. Effects of phosphoric acid concentration and etch duration on the shear bond strength of an orthodontic bonding resin to enamel (An in vitro study). Am J Orthod Dentofacial Orthop. 1989;96:485–92.
89. Shinchi MJ, Soma K, Nakabayashi N. The effect of phosphoric acid concentration on resin tag length and bond strength of a photo-cured resin to acid-etched enamel. Dent Mater. 2000;16: 324–9.

Prevention of Periodontal Deterioration/Damage

2

Abstract

This chapter emphasizes the reasons why lower incisors should generally not be proclined more than 2 mm since this orthodontic movement is associated with problems of *health*, *function*, *stability*, *and esthetics*. Facial movement of the teeth decreases the buccolingual thickness of the gingival tissue, which results in reduced height (recession) of the free gingival portion. In patients in whom the gingiva covering the labial of the lower incisors is thin and scalloped, orthodontic proclination of the lower incisors may cause not only gingival recession but also dehiscence. Both are examples of *health problems* associated with proclination of the incisors. An increase in the magnitude of the anterior open bite may occur in open-bite tendency malocclusions if lower incisors are moved labially and sometimes may even result in lip incompetence. These two are examples of *functional problems* associated with proclination of the incisors. There is evidence that post-retention *stability* of lower incisor alignment is compromised if the lower incisors were proclined during orthodontic treatment. Additionally, when the lower incisors are moved labially, facial *esthetics* could be compromised in pleasing facial profiles because as the teeth procline, the lips also move forward, while the chin stays back. An increase in lip protrusion could thus be associated with an undesirable appearance of a decreased chin projection and a diminished definition of the labiomental sulcus. Patient records are shown which illustrate the undesirable effects of lower incisor proclination. The contraindications for incisor proclination are discussed, and the orthodontic procedures recommended by the author to avoid incisor proclination in dentally crowded patients are shown.

2.1 Introduction

Several studies have compared the periodontal health between patients who had orthodontic treatment with individuals who did not have orthodontic treatment.

R. Justus, *Iatrogenic Effects of Orthodontic Treatment: Decision-Making in Prevention, Diagnosis, and Treatment*, DOI 10.1007/978-3-319-18353-4_2

Slutzkey and Levin [1] evaluated a cohort of 303 healthy patients who had routine dental examinations at a military dental center. They found increased gingival recession in young adults who had undergone orthodontic treatment (on average 4.8 years prior) compared to those who did not have orthodontic treatment. Also the severity and the extent of the recession were significantly correlated with past orthodontic treatment. This study supports the findings of systematic reviews that orthodontic treatment does not improve periodontal health and that it may actually make it worse.

Bollen et al. [2] carried out a systematic review of the relationship between orthodontic treatment and periodontal health. The conclusions were that patients with prior orthodontic treatment had 0.13-mm greater alveolar bone loss than patients without prior orthodontic treatment and that there were 0.23-mm greater pocket depth and 0.03-mm greater recession in subjects with prior orthodontic treatment. The reported small worsening of the periodontal conditions after orthodontic treatment was a generalized mean for the entire dentition. These small, yet significant, differences may be of clinical importance if it is a localized effect (a large worsening around a few teeth) rather than a generalized effect (small worsening around all teeth). This systematic review failed to find a beneficial effect of orthodontic treatment on periodontal health. On the contrary, patients with prior orthodontic care had greater alveolar bone loss, periodontal pocket depth, and gingival recession than individuals who had not received orthodontic treatment. These two studies [1, 2] suggest that orthodontists must be more careful in their treatment planning so as not to damage the gingival tissues.

In our practice of orthodontics, we have to decide, among many things, whether a patient requires extraction or non-extraction therapy. Non-extraction orthodontic therapy in patients who have reduced arch length requires arch expansion, frequently by moving incisors labially and posterior teeth laterally. Wennström [3] showed that facial movement of the teeth decreased the buccolingual thickness of the tissue, which resulted in gingival recession and an increased clinical crown height. In contrast, lingual movement increased the buccolingual thickness of the tissue, which resulted in coronal migration of the soft tissue margin and decreased clinical crown height. Thus, orthodontists might very well be putting patient's periodontal health at risk by expanding the arches.

Non-extraction therapy tends to move the incisors forward when dental crowding is present because arch perimeter has to be increased to be able to align the crowded teeth. In today's competitive world, orthodontists are frequently proclining the incisors to alleviate crowding, to treat patients with non-extraction therapy, even though extraction therapy may be indicated. In some instances, this may be the preference of the orthodontist, but often patients demand that treatment be done without extractions. The Internet has also made it easier for prospective patients to find out that orthodontists can treat patients with or without extractions. Patients naturally opt for non-extraction therapy, not understanding the negative consequences of incisor proclination. Orthodontists and orthodontic companies continue to introduce new ways of squeezing all teeth into dental arches, encroaching upon the enveloping muscular and periodontal equilibrium and filling the face and smiles with teeth to overflowing [4], regardless of the gingival health consequences. Proffit et al. [5] state that "……non-extraction treatment and expansion of the dental arches once again are being carried to an extreme."

There are, however, additional reasons why lower incisor proclination should generally be avoided. These are that lower incisor proclination:

- Increases the magnitude of the anterior open bite in open-bite tendency malocclusions
- Increases the probability of lip incompetence
- Compromises post-retention lower incisor alignment stability
- Diminishes chin prominence appearance as the lips are pushed forward

Clinical examples which illustrate the undesirable effects of lower incisor proclination are shown in the following subchapters as well as examples of the procedures the author recommends to avoid lower incisor proclination.

2.2 Apical Migration (Recession) of the Gingival Margin Associated with Lower Incisor Proclination

During the orthodontic treatment planning process, it is important for clinicians to appreciate that differences in gingival tissue architecture can affect treatment outcomes.

Two biotypes of gingival architecture have been described in the literature. These are thick-flat and thin-scalloped gingiva [6, 7]. Thick gingival tissue is probably the image most associated with periodontal health. The tissue is dense in appearance with a fairly large zone of attachment. The gingival topography is relatively flat with the suggestion of a thick underlying bony architecture. Surgical evaluation of these areas often reveals relatively thick underlying osseous forms. Thin gingival tissue tends to be delicate and almost translucent in appearance. The tissue appears friable with a minimal zone of attached gingiva. The soft tissue is highly accentuated and often suggestive of thin or minimal bone over the labial roots. Surgical evaluation often reveals thin labial bone with the possible presence of fenestration and dehiscence [8]. These two tissue biotypes have different gingival and osseous architectures exhibiting different responses when subjected to orthodontic tooth movements. These different responses dictate different treatment modalities. Evaluation of gingival tissue biotypes is thus important in orthodontic treatment planning. Since thick and thin gingival biotypes are associated with thick and thin osseous patterns, the two tissue types will respond differently.

Cook et al. [9] evaluated the correlation between labial plate thickness and thin or thick gingival biotypes—using information obtained from cone beam computed tomography, diagnostic impressions, and clinical examinations of maxillary anterior teeth—and concluded that a significant association existed between gingival biotype and labial plate thickness.

It has been shown that subjects with thin and vulnerable marginal tissue may be prone to the development of gingival recession due to orthodontic movement of the teeth away from the alveolar process [3, 10, 11]. Therefore, gingival biotype should be evaluated and taken into account during the treatment planning stage. A gingival thickness of 2 mm or more is defined as thick biotype, while a gingival thickness of 1.5 mm or less as thin biotype [12]. Various methods have been proposed to measure tissue thickness. De Rouck et al. [13] introduced a simple method to determine the gingival thickness based on the transparency of a periodontal probe through the gingival margin while probing the sulcus at the midfacial aspect of incisors. If the outline of the underlying periodontal probe could be seen through the gingival margin, it was categorized as thin; if not, it was categorized as thick. This method is minimally invasive and was found to be highly reproducible, with 85 % intra-examiner repeatability in a clinical trial of 100 periodontally healthy subjects [13]. In a population study, thick periodontal biotypes were found to be more prevalent (85 %) than thin-scalloped forms (15 %) [14].

Wennström et al. found no relationship between the initial width of the keratinized gingiva and the tendency for the development of gingival recession during orthodontic tooth movements in monkeys. However, they did find that it is the buccolingual thickness that determines gingival recession and attachment loss at sites with gingivitis during orthodontic treatment. In cases with thin gingiva caused by the prominent position of the teeth, there is no need for pre-orthodontic gingival augmentation procedures; the recession and bone dehiscence will decrease when the teeth are moved to a more proper position within the alveolar bone [15]. Wennström also found that the gingival tissue with little thickness in the presence of dental plaque is more susceptible to apical migration of connective tissue attachment with marginal gingiva, especially near the teeth under the influence of orthodontic force [16].

Thus, knowledge of the periodontal biotype is of fundamental importance because the anatomical characteristics of the periodontium, such as gingival thickness, gingival width, and alveolar bone morphology, will determine periodontal behavior when submitted to orthodontic treatment. It should be emphasized that tooth position can significantly alter the gingival parameters. Patients with thin-scalloped biotypes are considered at risk as they have been associated with a compromised soft tissue response following expansion orthodontic therapy [3].

It can be concluded that when the labial gingival tissue covering the lower incisors is of the thin-scalloped biotype, orthodontic proclination of these teeth could result in a reduction of gingival height and perhaps also gingival dehiscence. Patient A illustrates the latter problem. This patient had thin-scalloped labial gingiva covering her lower incisors (Figs. 2.1, 2.2, 2.3, and 2.6). She developed a gingival dehiscence on the labial of her mandibular left central incisor root during her orthodontic treatment (Fig. 2.17). This gingival defect probably arose due to the orthodontic proclination of the lower incisors, which was required for a successful mandibular surgical setback.

Patient A was a 19.8-year-old healthy female with a bilateral Class III malocclusion (Figs. 2.1, 2.2, and 2.3). A family history of prognathism was reported.

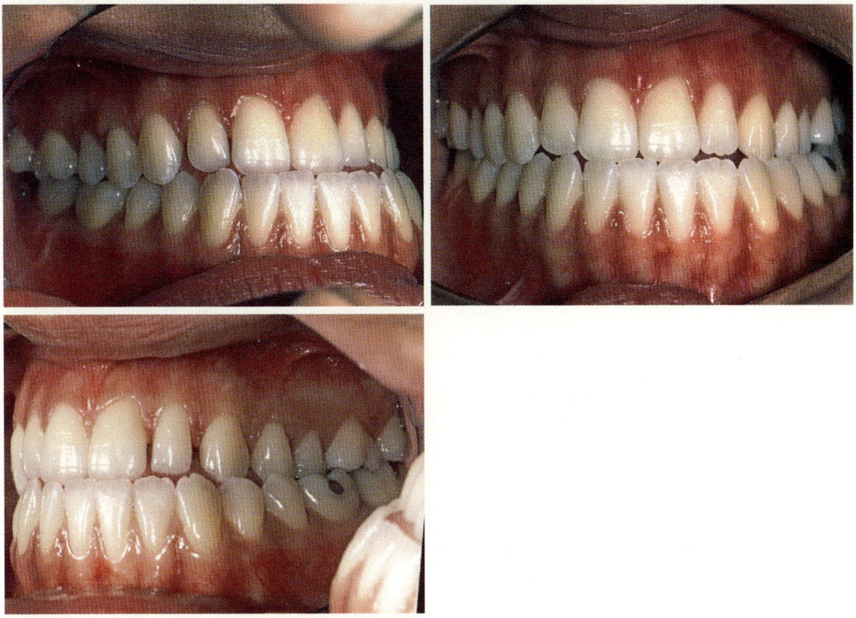

Figs. 2.1, 2.2, and 2.3 Pretreatment intraoral views. Note Class III molar and canine relationship, mandibular midline shift to the left, maxillary left canine and premolars in lingual cross-bite, and anterior cross-bite (visible on the extreme lower right side of Fig. 2.3). Note narrow maxillary lateral incisors and thin-scalloped gingival biotype with almost transparent gingiva covering the incisor roots

Her facial profile was prognathic (Fig. 2.4) with both her lower lip and chin appearing more prominent in relation to the rest of her soft tissue profile. Her cephalometric lateral headfilm (Fig. 2.5) demonstrated an ANB angle of 0.5° (SNA 85°, SNB 84.5°); her Wits appraisal of jaw disharmony was a negative 9 mm, and her mandibular plane angle relative to the SN line was 34°; her lower incisors were retroclined relative to her mandibular plane (81°); they were 6-mm forward of the NB line, and her maxillary incisors were 4-mm forward of the NA line and at 106° relative to the SN line; she had a negative 3-mm overjet (Fig. 2.6), with all maxillary incisors in anterior crossbite and with minimal overbite. There was 3 mm of mandibular dental crowding (Fig. 2.7) and 4 mm of dental spacing in the maxillary arch mainly due to narrow lateral incisors (Fig. 2.8), which resulted in a tooth size discrepancy. In the transverse relationship, the mandible had a 2-mm shift to the left (Fig. 2.9) due to the fact that the maxillary left canine and left premolars were in lingual crossbite (Figs. 2.2 and 2.3). In centric occlusion, the mandibular dental midline was 2 mm to the left of both the maxillary dental and the facial midlines due to a mandibular forced shift from centric relation to centric occlusion (Fig. 2.2). The frontal face view shows her mandible shifted to the left side while in centric occlusion (Fig. 2.9), but symmetric while smiling and out of occlusion (Fig. 2.10).

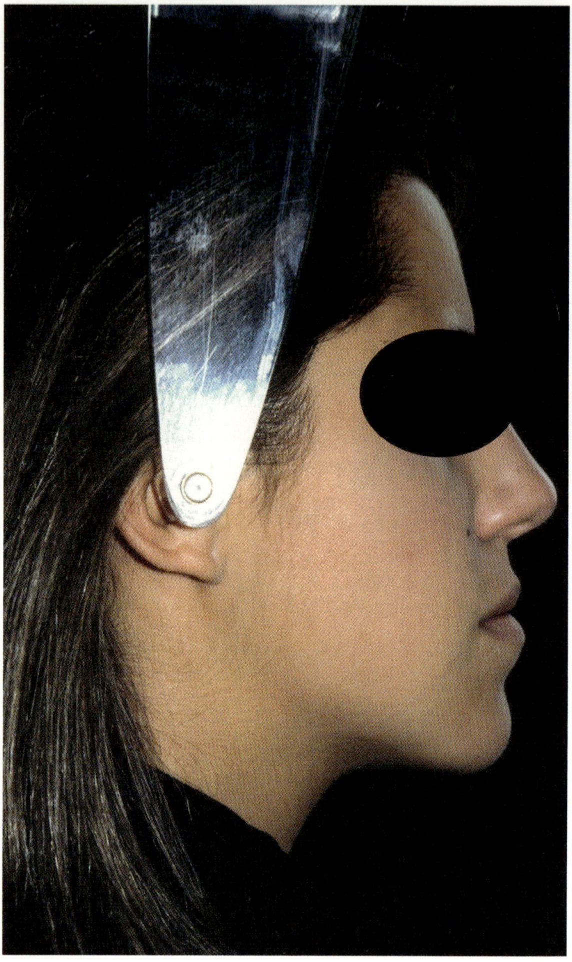

Fig. 2.4 Pretreatment profile facial photograph. Note Class III facial profile

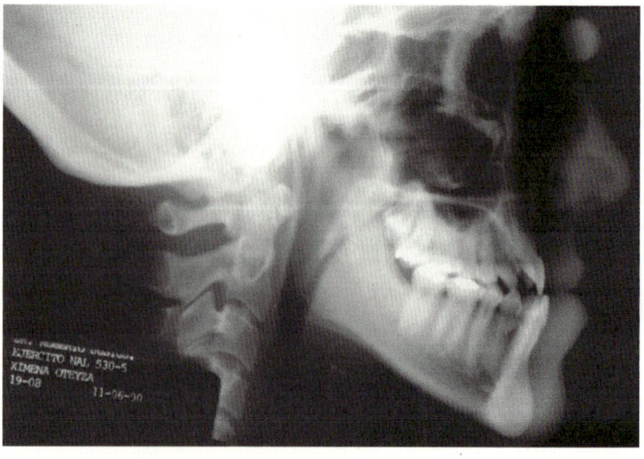

Fig. 2.5 Pretreatment cephalogram. Note anterior crossbite associated with a Class III skeletal relationship

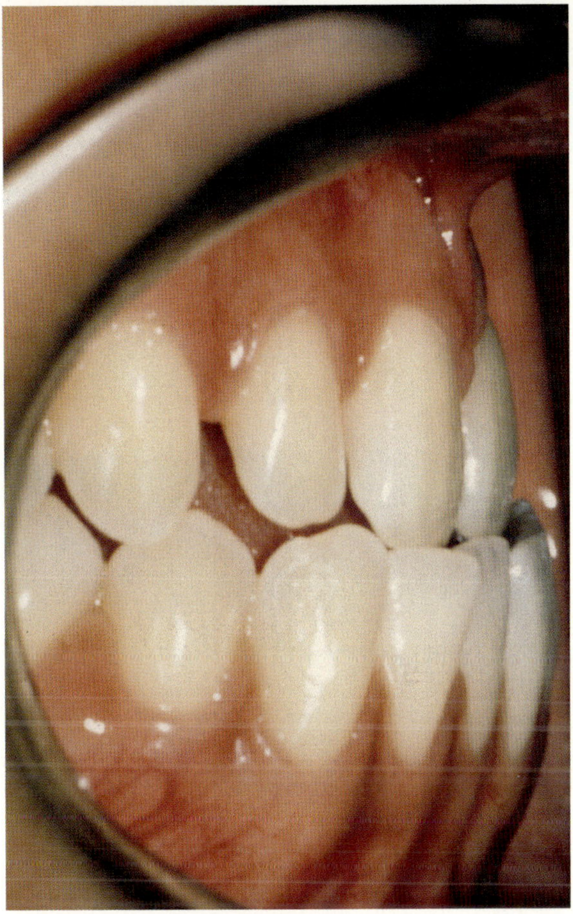

Fig. 2.6 Pretreatment lateral intraoral view of incisors in anterior crossbite. Note narrow maxillary lateral incisor and thin-scalloped gingival biotype

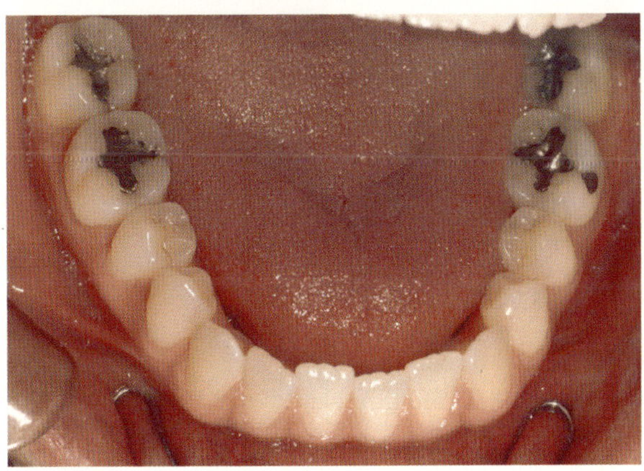

Fig. 2.7 Pretreatment occlusal view of the lower arch. Note 3 mm of dental crowding

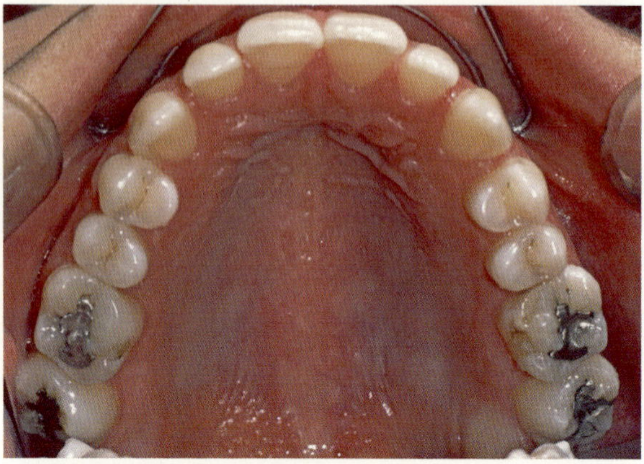

Fig. 2.8 Pretreatment occlusal view of the upper arch. Note dental spacing mesial and distal to the lateral incisors and distal to the left canine, totaling 4 mm

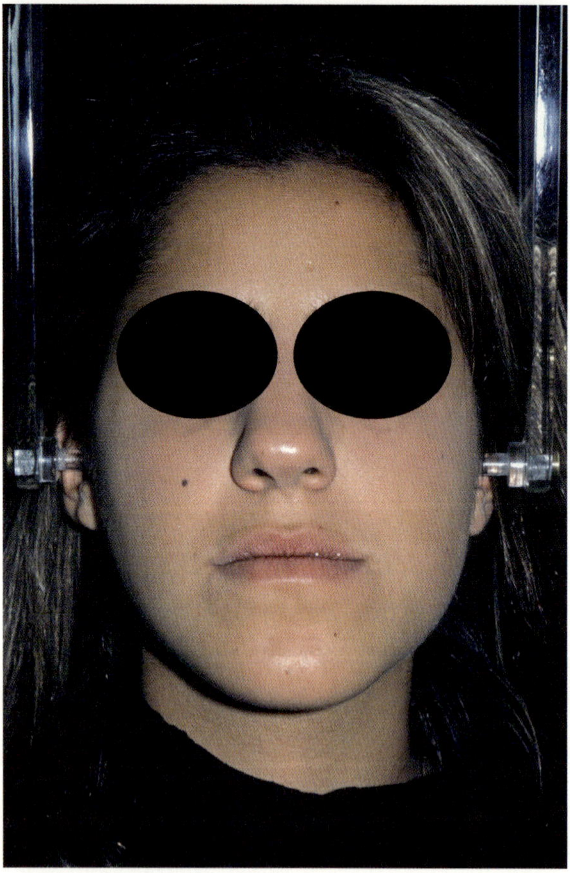

Fig. 2.9 Pretreatment frontal facial view with the teeth in occlusion. Note the chin deviated toward the left side

The patient and her parents were informed that extraction of the two mandibular first premolars, combined with orthodontic treatment, might correct both the anterior and the posterior crossbites but that with this extraction therapy, the chin

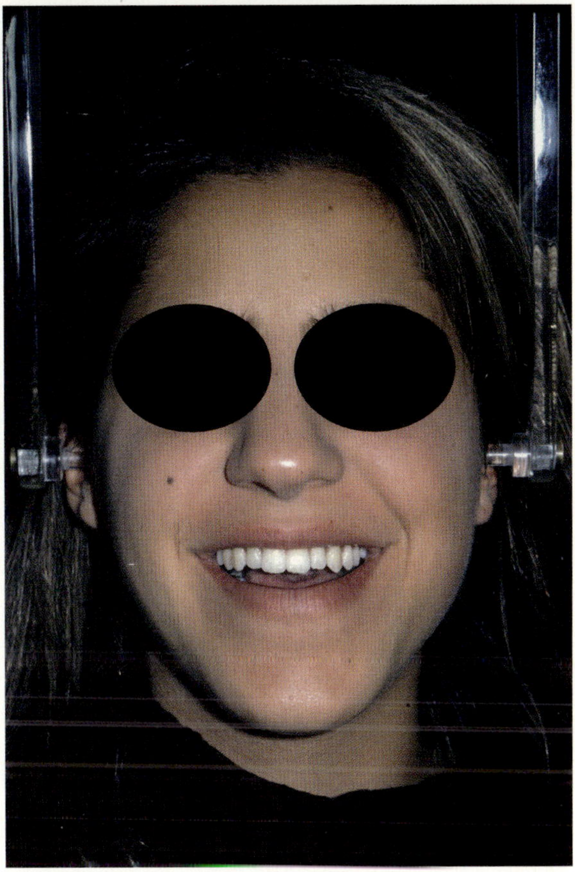

Fig. 2.10 Pretreatment frontal facial view with the teeth out of occlusion. Note that the chin is less deviated toward the left

prominence would appear increased because the lower lip would be retracted and the retroclined lower incisors would appear even more so (observe extreme right side of Fig. 2.3). Non-extraction orthodontic therapy combined with a mandibular surgical setback was thus recommended.

The treatment objectives were to align the lower teeth, to close the maxillary spaces by bonding composite buildups on the narrow maxillary lateral incisors, and to surgically setback her mandible to reduce the excessive chin projection while simultaneously correcting both the anterior and the posterior crossbites. The left posterior crossbite would be automatically corrected during the mandibular surgical setback because as the mandible is surgically moved backward, its transverse width diminishes. Both the patient and her parents accepted this treatment plan, except for the maxillary lateral incisor composite buildups. Thus, the treatment plan was modified. It included closing all maxillary spaces, by incisor retroclination, and aligning the lower teeth, by lower incisor proclination. These orthodontic movements would result in an increased negative overjet thereby creating greater surgical space to achieve facial harmony. This increased negative overjet would allow the surgeon to maximize the mandibular surgical setback and thereby diminish the excessive chin prominence.

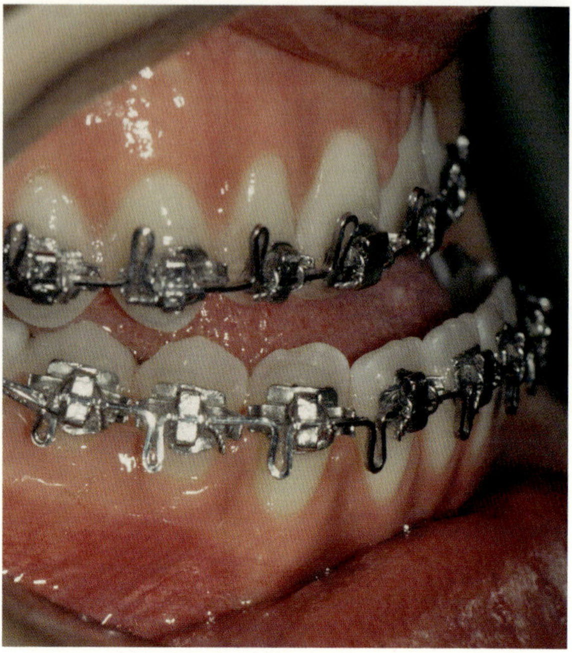

Fig. 2.11 Progress presurgical lateral intraoral view of incisors in anterior crossbite. Note that the negative overjet has been increased, that all maxillary spaces have been closed, and that surgical orthodontic arch wires are in place

Full brackets were bonded to both dental arches, and a progression of arch wires were tied to all the brackets. Six months later, an increased negative overjet of 10 mm had been created (Fig. 2.11) by proclining the lower incisors from 6 to 8.5 mm relative to the NB line and by retroclining the maxillary incisors from 4 to 0 mm relative to the NA line. The thin-scalloped labial gingiva covering the lower incisors is noticeable (Figs. 2.6 and 2.11) and also the worsening of her facial profile, due to proclination of her lower incisors and retroclination of her upper incisors (Fig. 2.12). Full orthodontic records were taken at this time, including a lateral headfilm (Fig. 2.13). Surgical orthodontic arch wires were tied to the brackets (Fig. 2.11), and a chin cup appliance (Fig. 2.14) was given to her to be used nighttime during the 6 months following surgery. The purpose of this appliance was to minimize the relapse tendency of the mandible to move forward again, as reported by Proffit et al. [17]. These authors suggested that the anterior relapse tendency of the mandible could be due to muscular pull as function resumes and that the altered orientation of the elevator muscles, which occurs when the mandible is moved posteriorly, could lead to some forward adjustment of the mandible particularly if the ramus was pushed to a more vertical inclination during surgery. Thus, the chin cup appliance may help stabilize the mandible while postsurgical muscle adaptation takes place.

The patient underwent surgical setback of her mandible, with simultaneous extraction of her maxillary third molars (Fig. 2.15). One month postsurgery, the facial profile appears greatly improved (Fig. 2.16). Unfortunately, a labial gingival dehiscence developed following the surgical procedure. The dehiscence partially

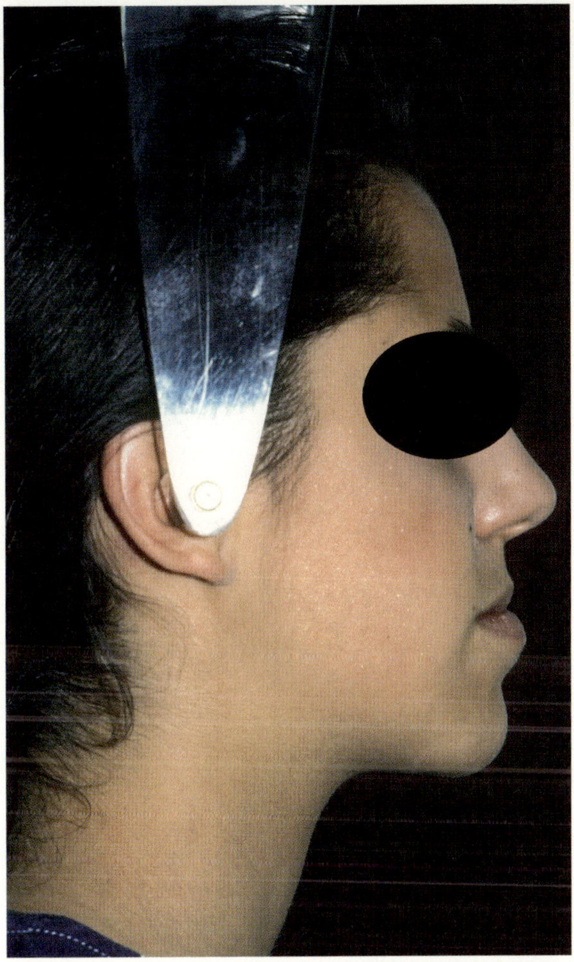

Fig. 2.12 Presurgical facial profile view. Note worsening of the Class III profile due to the orthodontic proclination of the lower incisors and the retroclination of the upper incisors

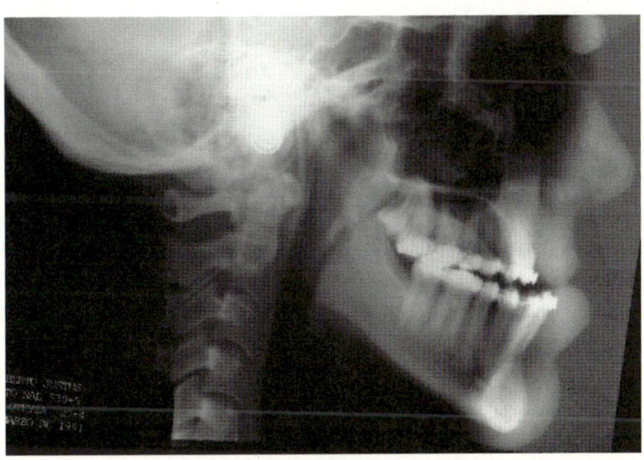

Fig. 2.13 Presurgical cephalogram. Note orthodontic incisor decompensation created in preparation for mandibular surgical setback

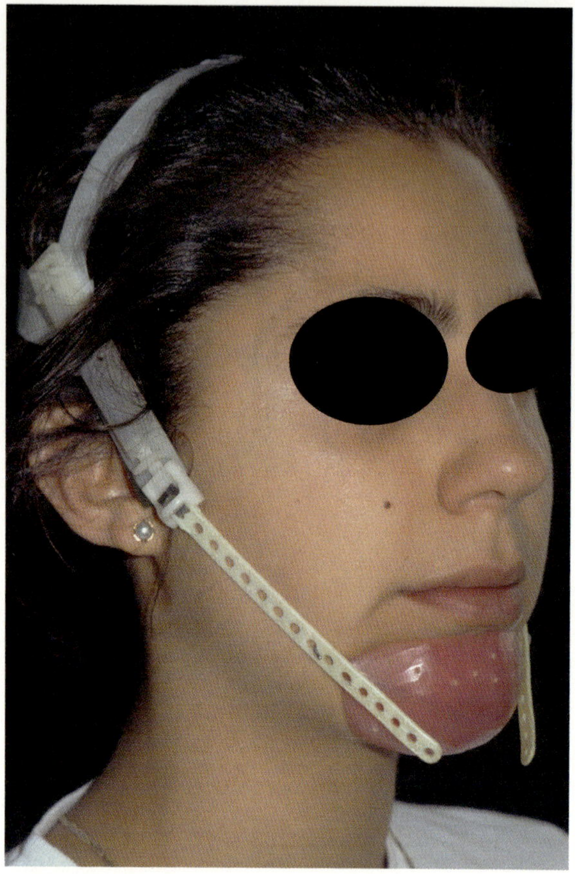

Fig. 2.14 Chin cup appliance given to the patient to minimize the postsurgical relapse tendency of the mandible to move forward again due to muscle pull

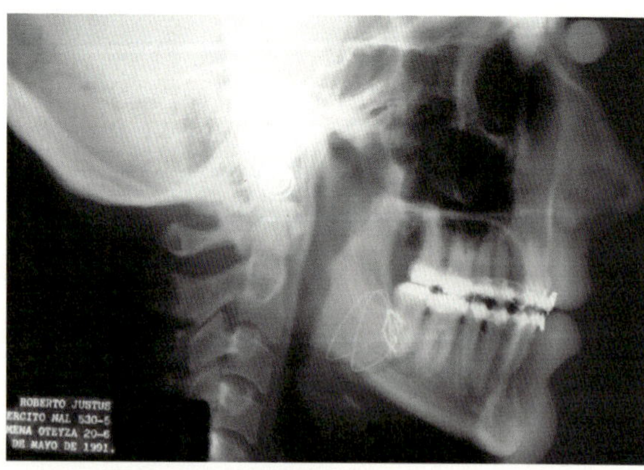

Fig. 2.15 Immediate postsurgery lateral cephalogram. Note normal skeletal and dental relationships

denuded the mandibular left central incisor root. The author attributes the development of this dehiscence to two reasons. The first is that the patient did not brush her teeth well following the surgical procedure, as is usually the case in orthognathic

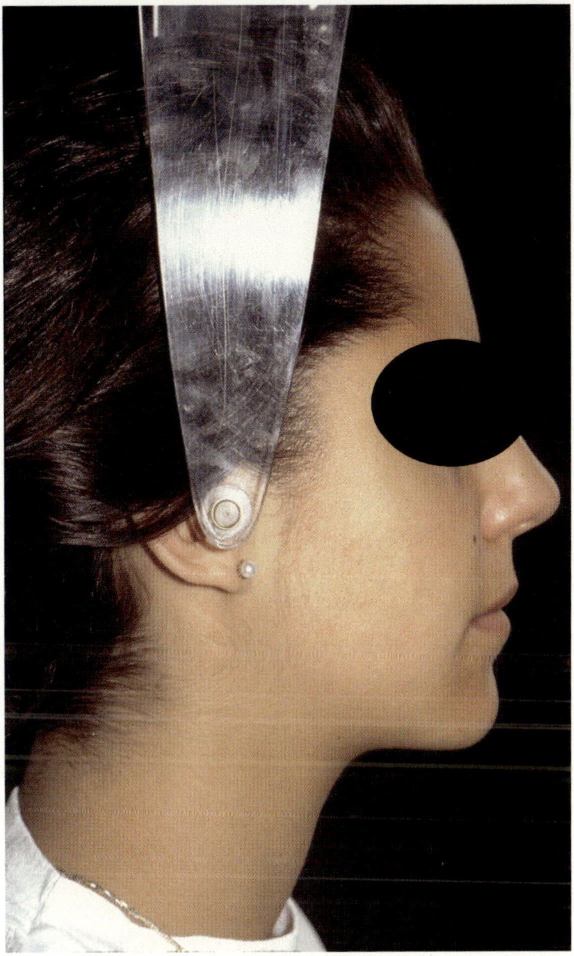

Fig. 2.16 One month postsurgery facial profile view. Note pleasing facial features

surgery patients; the second is that the patient's gingival biotype was thin scalloped, which is more susceptible to suffer dehiscence when combined with incisor proclination [3, 16]. The patient was asked to maintain the cleanliness of this area. Three months postsurgery, the brackets were removed, removable orthodontic retainers were given, and posttreatment records were obtained. The patient was then referred to a periodontist to cover the dehiscence (Fig. 2.17) with a free gingival graft (Fig. 2.18), which was harvested from her palatal mucosa.

The patient and her parents were very pleased with both the orthodontic (Figs. 2.19, 2.20, 2.21, 2.22, and 2.23) and the facial results (Figs. 2.24, 2.25, and 2.26); facial profile improvement was indeed dramatic when one compares the pre- and the posttreatment facial profile photographs (Figs. 2.4 and 2.24) because the chin and the lower lip projection decreased. The posttreatment cephalometric lateral headfilm (Fig. 2.27) demonstrates an excellent maxillo-mandibular relationship, as well as adequate cephalometric incisor positions. Her ANB angle is now 4°

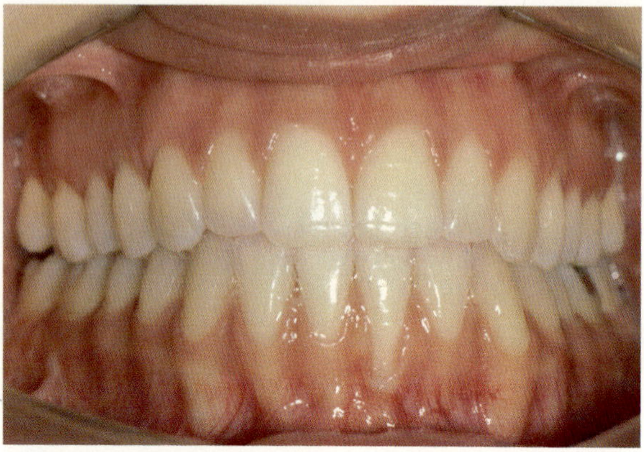

Fig. 2.17 Posttreatment intraoral frontal view. Observe gingival dehiscence in the lower left central incisor root area with partial root denudation

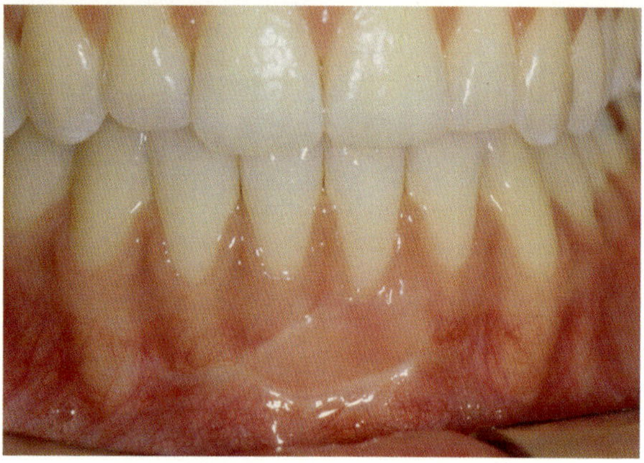

Fig. 2.18 Posttreatment intraoral photograph taken after a free gingival graft was placed to cover the dehiscence. Graft was harvested from the patient's palatal mucosa

(SNA 84° and SNB 80°), and her Wits appraisal is a positive 2 mm. Incisor positions are also within the cephalometric norms, allowing the lips and chin to have a normal position. Her lower incisors, which were originally retroclined relative to her mandibular plane at 81°, are now at 88°. These incisors were 6 mm in front of the NB line and are now again at 6 mm; her maxillary incisors changed from being 4 mm to 2 mm in front of the NA line and from 107° to 90° with respect to the SN line. These slightly retropositioned maxillary incisors were the result of having closed the maxillary spaces orthodontically. A better occlusal result could have been achieved had the maxillary spaces been closed with lateral incisor composite buildups. With buildups, the maxillary incisors would be more proclined, allowing the mandible to be more advanced, with cusps coinciding with embrasures.

A maxillary and a mandibular removable retainer were given to the patient one day after bracket debonding with instructions to wear them nighttime for as long as she wished to have straight teeth. The upper retainer that the author recommends is the wraparound type (Fig. 2.28). The reason for using this type of retainer is that the labial/buccal wire does not interfere with the occlusion. The lower retainer design

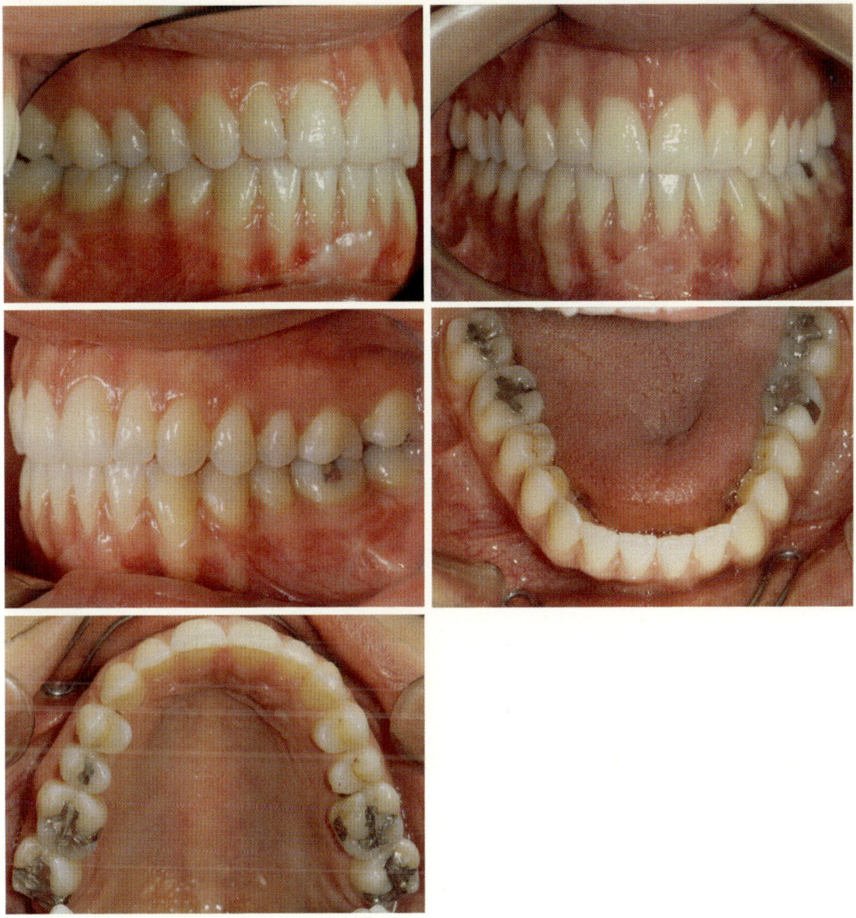

Figs. 2.19, 2.20, 2.21, 2.22, and 2.23 Posttreatment intraoral views. Note well-aligned teeth but not in an ideal Class I occlusion due to the tooth size discrepancy arising from narrow maxillary lateral incisors

can be seen in Fig. 2.29. It is a retainer that covers both the labial and the lingual of all the teeth in the arch. These retainers impede labiolingual and rotational tooth movements from occurring and also prevent spaces from reopening [18]. Figures 2.30 and 2.31 show the retainers in place. The gingival-labial acrylic of the lower retainer has been cut away in the grafted area. The patient was instructed to return for annual retainer checkups.

In hind sight, a preventative gingival graft should have been placed prior to orthodontic treatment to increase the gingival thickness on the labial of the lower incisors. The patient originally had thin-scalloped labial gingiva covering the lower incisor area, which the author failed to act upon. Proclination of the lower incisors was required to decompensate the lower incisors in preparation for orthognathic surgery. However, periodontal health in the lower incisor region was jeopardized in

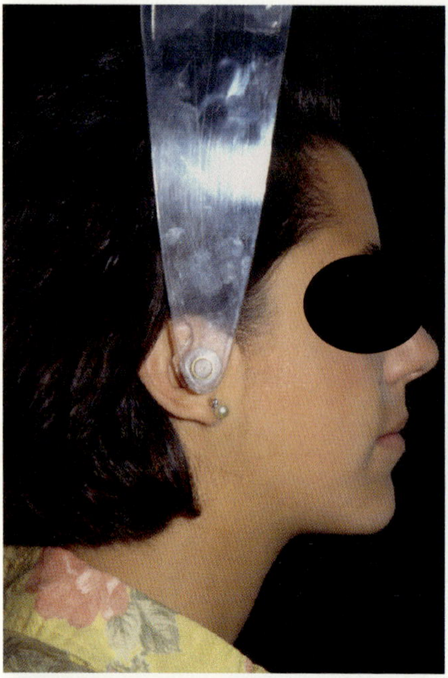

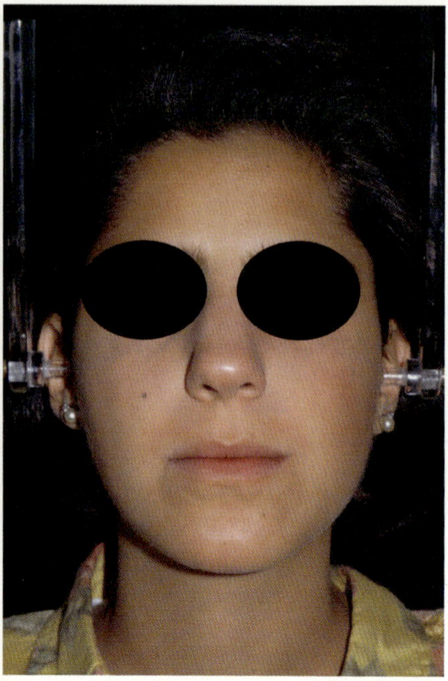

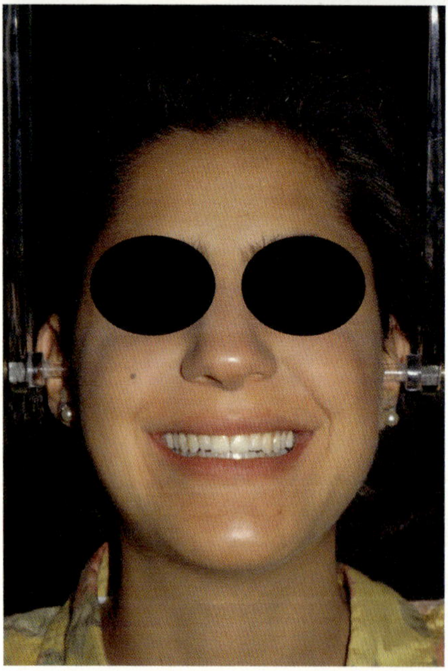

Figs. 2.24, 2.25, and 2.26 Posttreatment facial views. Note facial harmony

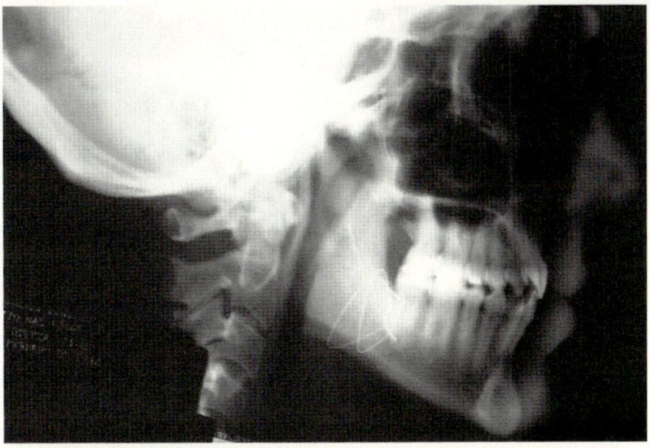

Fig. 2.27 Posttreatment cephalogram. Note normal overjet and pleasing facial profile

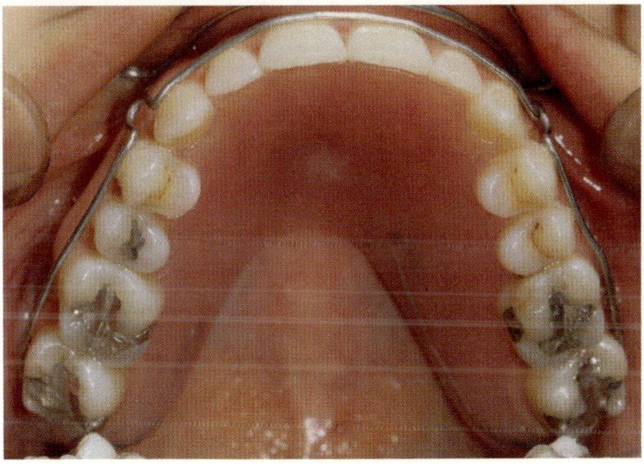

Fig. 2.28 Intraoral occlusal view of the removable maxillary wraparound retainer

this patient by having proclined the lower incisors without prior placement of a preventative soft tissue graft. Orthodontists should remember that a Hippocratic orthodontic practice means that patients end up healthier dentally and *periodontally* after orthodontic treatment or at the very least that patients maintain their initial oral tissue health in spite of undergoing orthodontic treatment.

2.3 Increase in the Magnitude of Anterior Open Bite Associated with Lower Incisor Proclination

Orthodontic proclination of incisors in a patient with a pretreatment anterior open bite could result in an increase in the magnitude of the anterior open bite. This is due to the drawbridge effect (Fig. 2.32). This effect occurs because as the incisors are proclined, they rotate in such a manner that the incisor borders move away from the occlusal plane (Figs. 2.33 and 2.34) creating a frank anterior open bite.

Patient B is presented to illustrate the worsening of an anterior open bite in a patient whose incisors were orthodontically proclined. This patient clearly demonstrates the association between the drawbridge effect and anterior open bite.

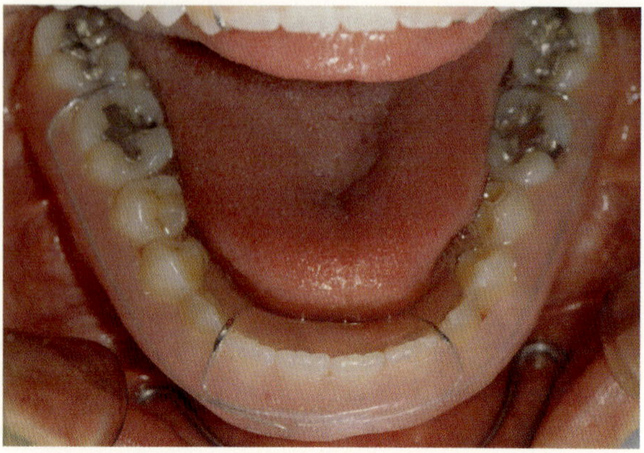

Fig. 2.29 Intraoral occlusal view of the removable mandibular retainer

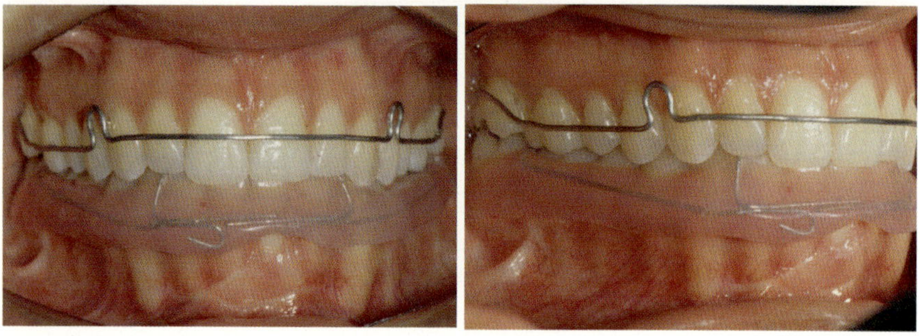

Figs. 2.30 and 2.31 Intraoral frontal and right lateral views with retainers in place. Note that in the mandibular retainer, the gingival-labial acrylic has been cut away in the area corresponding to the graft so as not to impinge on it

This patient illustrates that non-extraction treatment in the presence of a 3-mm mandibular and maxillary arch length deficiency led to serious and undesired consequences. Specifically, the patient suffered an increase in the magnitude of a pre-existing anterior open bite and also an increase in lip protrusion, with the lower lip that is too protrusive relative to the soft tissue chin creating an unattractive labiomental sulcus. This is an example of what may occur with non-extraction treatment in a case that should have been treated with extractions based on the facial features and on the degree of arch length deficiency present.

When a patient exhibits a pretreatment anterior open bite, even if there is minor dental crowding, the open bite worsens if the incisors are proclined with non-extraction therapy. The following case report of patient B illustrates this.

Patient B was a 17.3-year-old healthy female with a Class I malocclusion (Figs. 2.35, 2.36, and 2.37) with 3 mm of dental crowding in both mandibular and maxillary arches (Figs. 2.38 and 2.39). The patient had a 2-mm anterior open bite on her right central maxillary incisor and a 1-mm open bite on her left central maxillary incisor, and the rest of her incisors exhibited no open bite but had insufficient overbite (Figs. 2.35 and 2.37). She had anterior overjet of 5 mm on her maxillary

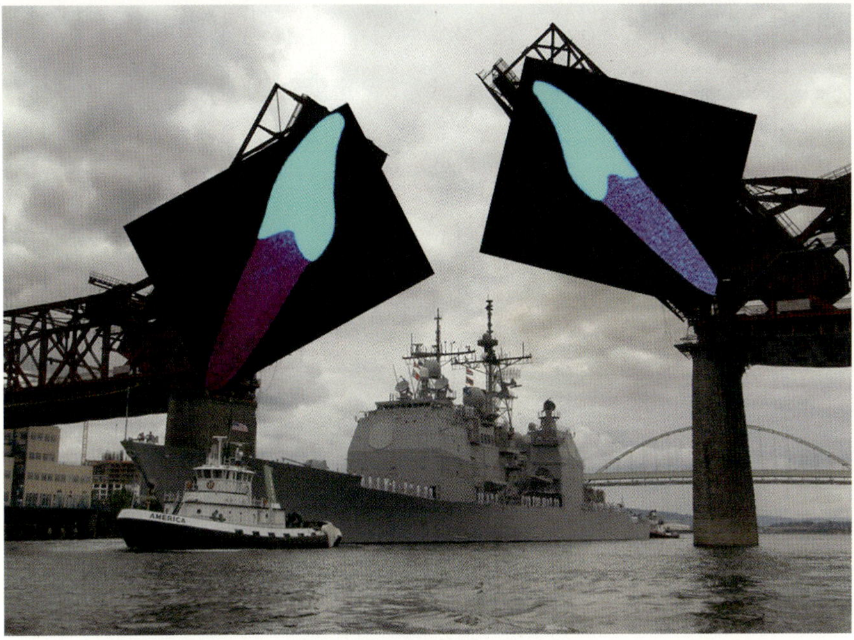

Fig. 2.32 Drawbridge effect

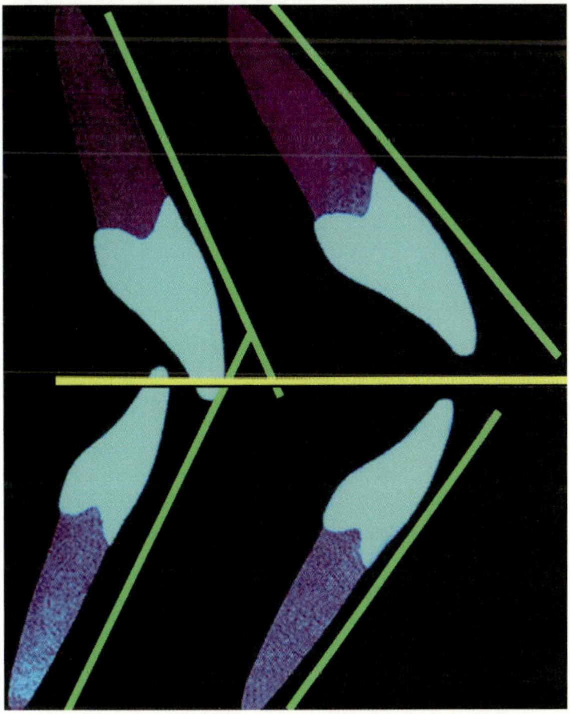

Fig. 2.33 Drawbridge effect. Observe that as the incisors are proclined, the further away their incisal borders distance themselves from the occlusal plane

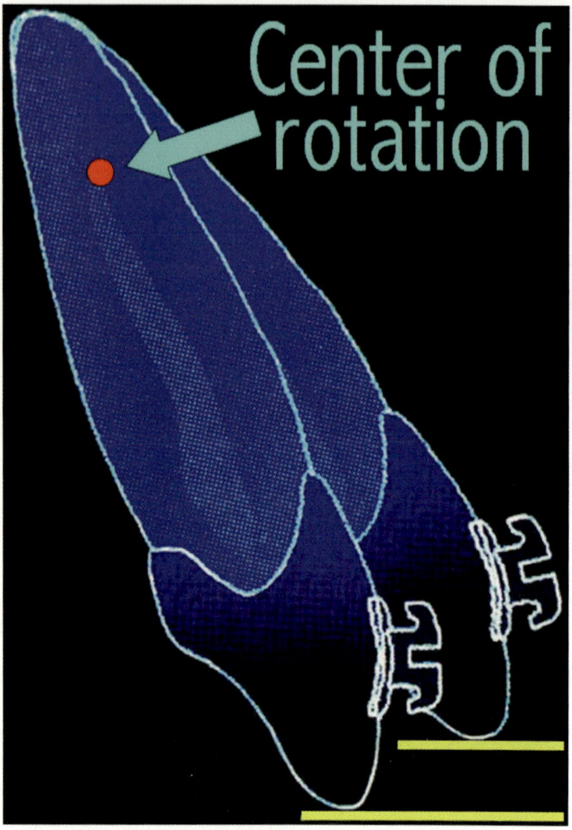

Fig. 2.34 Drawbridge effect. Observe how the maxillary incisors rotate away from the original occlusal plane as they are proclined

right central incisor. Her ANB was 6° (SNA 79°, SNB 73°), and she had a steep mandibular plane angle of 50° relative to the SN line (Fig. 2.40). She had a long face syndrome (Fig. 2.41) exhibiting a convex profile, lower lip protrusion, a deficient chin prominence, labiomental sulcus with poor definition, short neck-chin distance, and elongated lower lip which was incompetent. Her lower incisors were 16 mm in front of the NB line and 102° relative to the mandibular plane, and her maxillary incisors were 8 mm in front of the NA line and 113° relative to the SN line (Fig. 2.40)

The patient was treated with full fixed appliances for 4 months by an orthodontist who used a non-extraction orthodontic protocol to correct the dental alignment (Figs. 2.42 and 2.43). Space to align the teeth was created by interproximal reduction (stripping) and by expanding the arches, which included proclining the incisors. The patient's father and his family were then transferred to another country by the company he worked for. The patient came to the author's office with the request from the original orthodontist to close the anterior open bite.

A greater anterior open bite had developed (Figs. 2.44, 2.45, and 2.46) as a consequence of the non-extraction therapy. This can be observed by comparing the pretreatment intraoral photographs (Figs. 2.35, 2.36, and 2.37) to the progress

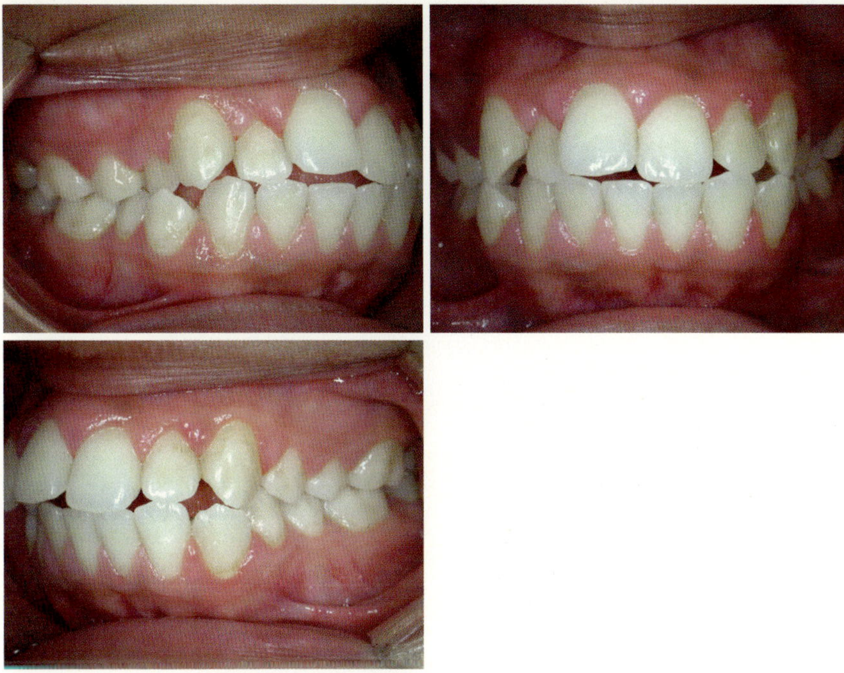

Figs. 2.35, 2.36, and 2.37 Pretreatment intraoral views with teeth in occlusion. Observe a 2-mm anterior open bite of the maxillary right central incisor and insufficient overbite of the rest of the incisors

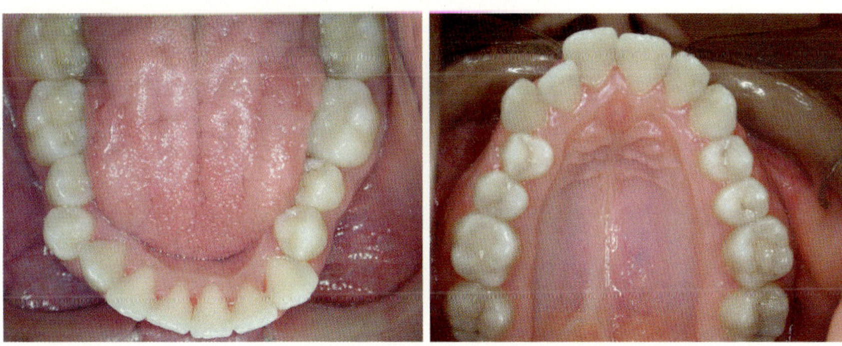

Figs. 2.38 and 2.39 Pretreatment mandibular and maxillary intraoral occlusal views. Observe a 3-mm arch length deficiency in both arches

intraoral photographs (Figs. 2.44, 2.45, and 2.46), as well as the initial cephalogram (Fig. 2.40) to the progress cephalogram (Fig. 2.47). Due to the non-extraction orthodontic treatment, the lower incisors were proclined from an initial 16 to 16.5 mm relative to the NB line. The maxillary incisors were proclined from 8 to 10 mm relative to the NA line. The consequence of these proclinations was a worsening of the

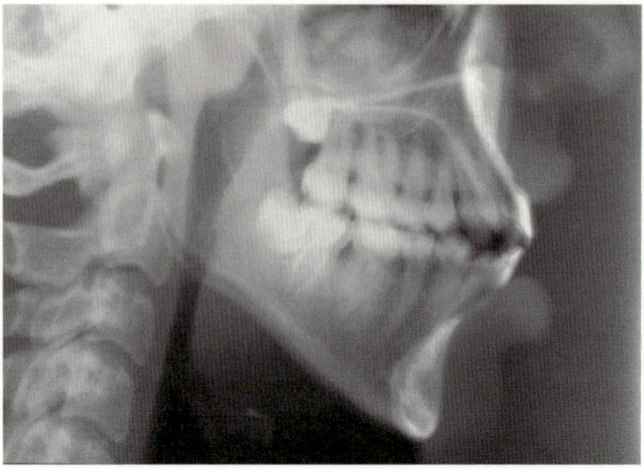

Fig. 2.40 Pretreatment lateral cephalogram. Note proclined lower incisors (16 mm in front of the NB line and 102° relative to the mandibular plane) and proclined maxillary incisors (8 mm in front of the NA line and 113° relative to the SN line). Also note a very steep mandibular plane (50° to the SN line) and a 2-mm anterior open bite of the right maxillary central incisor while the left maxillary central incisor has insufficient overbite

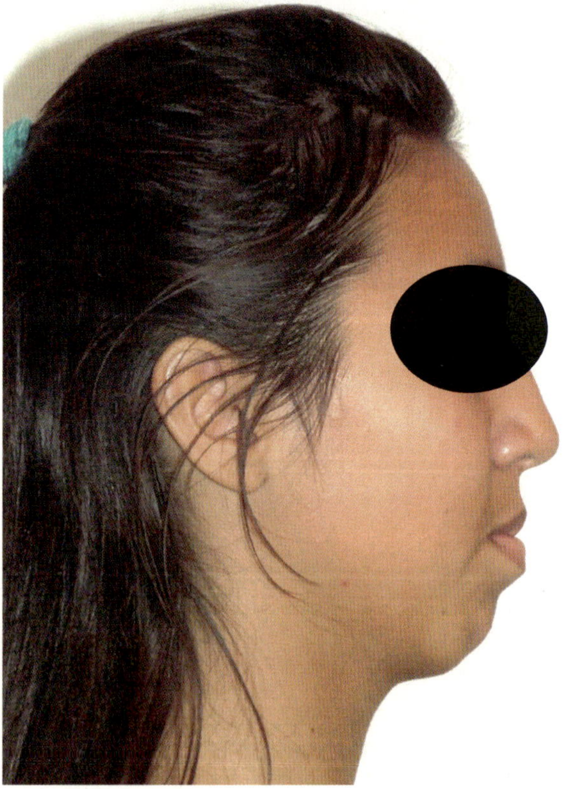

Fig. 2.41 Pretreatment facial profile view. Note long face syndrome with convex profile, lower lip protrusion, a deficient chin prominence, labiomental sulcus with poor definition, short neck-chin distance, and incompetent elongated lower lip

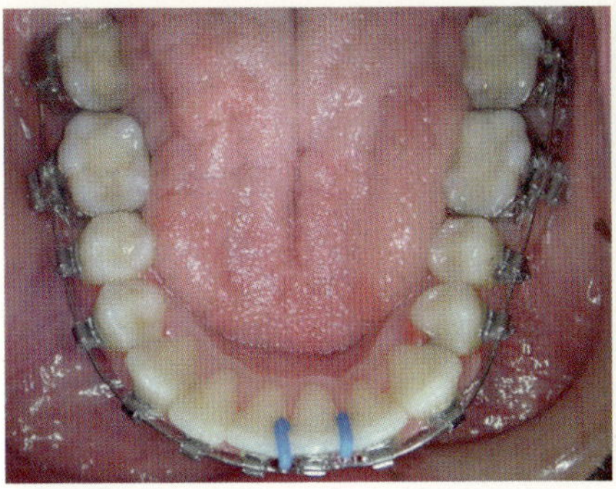

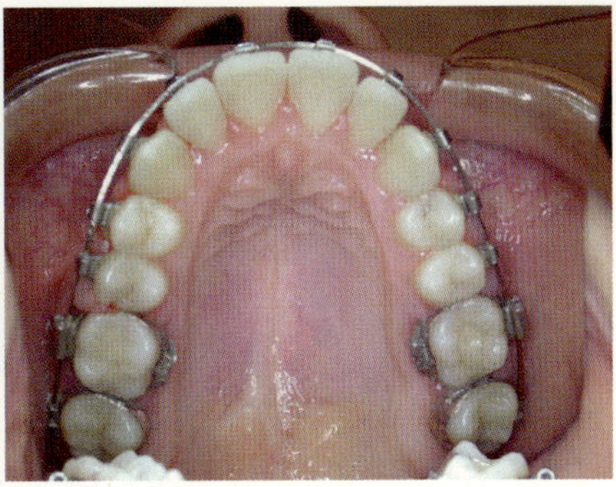

Figs. 2.42 and 2.43 Progress mandibular and maxillary intraoral occlusal views after 4 months of orthodontic treatment. Observe resolution of the dental crowding using full fixed appliances with a non-extraction treatment which included increasing arch length and interproximal reduction of teeth. Blue Alastik separators placed between incisors to create space for alignment

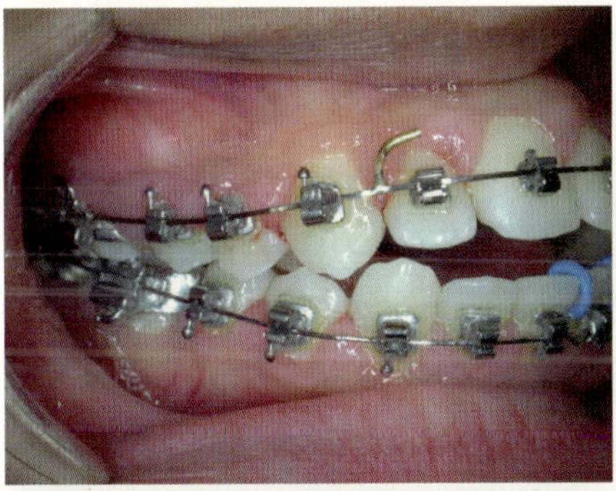

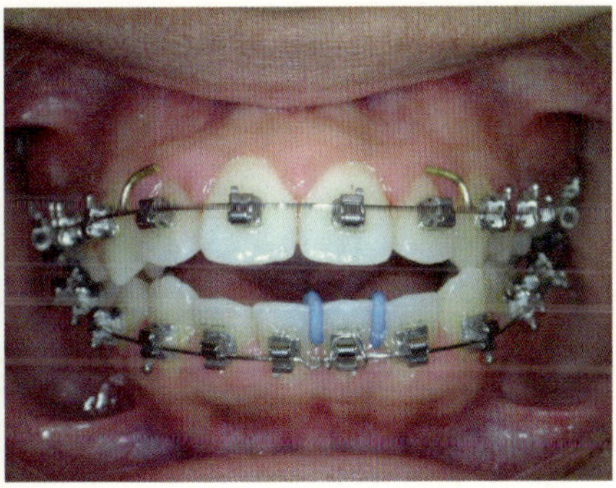

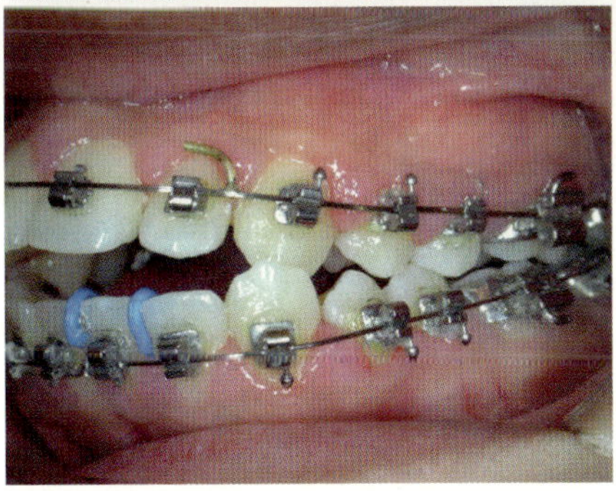

Figs. 2.44, 2.45, and 2.46 Progress intraoral views with teeth in occlusion, after 4 months of orthodontic treatment. Observe increase in the magnitude of the anterior open bite

original open bite due to the drawbridge effect. Initially, the open bite appeared only on the maxillary central incisors (Figs. 2.35, 2.36, and 2.37). However, the progress photographs show all incisors with a 4-mm open bite (Figs. 2.44, 2.45, and 2.46). As the maxillary incisors were proclined, they rotated moving their incisal borders

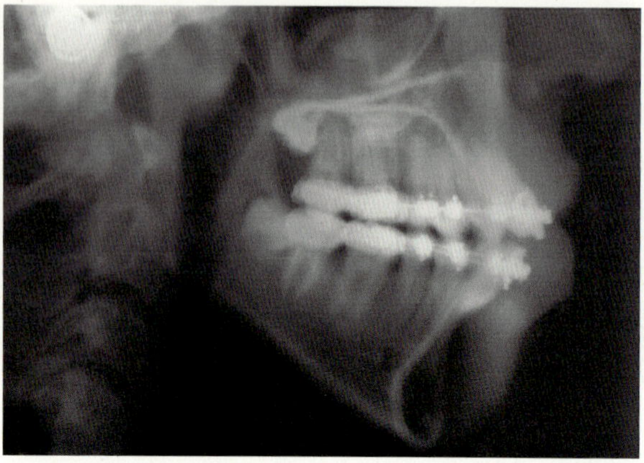

Fig. 2.47 Progress lateral cephalogram. Note a greater magnitude of anterior open bite developed due to the drawbridge effect associated with proclination of incisors. Note that both mandibular and particularly maxillary incisors were proclined

away from the occlusal plane, thus opening the bite. Note that in the initial cephalogram (Fig. 2.40), the incisal border of the right maxillary central incisor is 2 mm above the incisal border of the contralateral incisor, while the lateral incisors exhibit no open bite. Another negative consequence of having proclined the incisors, in addition to the worsening of the anterior open bite, was a further deterioration of the initial facial profile: increased lip protrusion (compare Figs. 2.41 and 2.48), more elongated lower lip, appearance of a more retrusive chin, and a diminished labiomental sulcus. Superimpositions of cranial base, maxilla, and mandible were not possible in this patient because the pretreatment and the progress lateral headfilms were not taken with the same machine.

Non-extraction treatment in the presence of even minor arch length deficiency, such as patient B exhibited, led to serious and undesired consequences, specifically increased magnitude of the preexisting anterior open bite and diminished facial attractiveness. This patient is an example of what may occur with non-extraction treatment in a "clear-cut" extraction case (based on facial features and lack of sufficient arch length). The original orthodontic treatment plan for patient B should have included therapy with premolar extractions combined with orthognathic surgery. The tendency for incisor irregularity relapse post-retention will probably be greater in patient B since there is now increased lingual pressure against the incisors due to their having been proclined against the lips. The following section addresses this issue.

2.4 Poor Post-retention Stability of Lower Incisor Alignment Associated with Lower Incisor Proclination

Evidence shows that proclination of lower incisors has a negative impact on long-term post-retention alignment stability. Orthodontists have known for a long time that mandibular incisors are the teeth that have the least post-retention stability. The University of Washington Graduate Orthodontic Department has for many years investigated the long-term post-retention stability of various orthodontic treatment

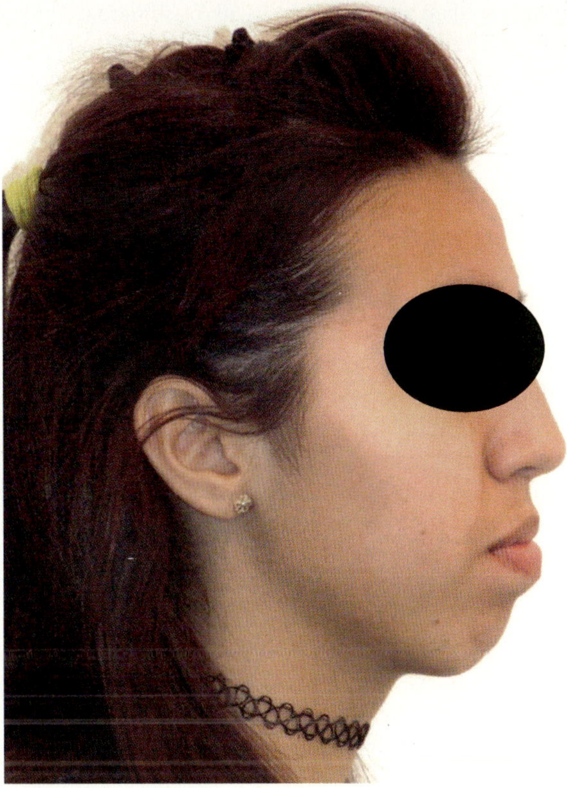

Fig. 2.48 Progress facial profile after 4 months of treatment. Note increased lip protrusion with the chin appearing less prominent relative to the lower lip (which elongated more) and even less definition of the labiomental sulcus

protocols. The studies evaluated groups of patients who were treated with various extraction patterns to correct dental crowding. The groups studied included the following extraction patterns: four first bicuspids [19–21], maxillary first and mandibular second bicuspids [22], and maxillary first bicuspids and mandibular incisors [23]. Long-term post-retention stability of non-extraction therapy was also investigated in patients who had generalized spacing [24] and in patients in whom mandibular arch length was increased in the mixed dentition [25].

Little et al. [25] studied a non-extraction group of 26 patients in the mixed dentition in which some crowding was present but not enough to justify extraction therapy. The research was carried out to answer the question whether there would be greater relapse using non-extraction therapy when mandibular arch length is increased during the mixed dentition to resolve crowding, compared with groups of patients treated with various extraction patterns to resolve dental crowding. The inclusion criteria for the non-extraction sample included a minimum increase of 1 mm in arch length during mixed dentition treatment, successful alignment results, and availability of full orthodontic records (pretreatment, posttreatment, and a minimum of 6 years post-retention). The researchers found that treating patients using a non-extraction approach, by increasing arch length during the mixed dentition, was the therapy that had the greatest incisor irregularity post-retention relapse of all the groups studied at the University of Washington. Thus, the author of this book suggests we pay heed to Dr. Little's quote, "expand the mandibular arch at your own risk" [26].

Another long-term post-retention study carried out in Nijmegen University (the Netherlands) confirms the lack of stability of mandibular alignment [27]. The available data suggest that moving lower incisors forward more than 2 mm is problematic for stability, probably because lip pressure seems to increase sharply at about that point [5]. Thus, in general, orthodontists should try to avoid non-extraction therapy in patients who have moderate to severe dental crowding because the post-retention relapse will be greater and also because of the many additional issues associated with lower incisor proclination mentioned previously.

Dr. Little [26] states "........ for both treated and untreated cases, arch length and width reduction occurs from the mixed dentition stage into the teen-age years, and to a lesser degree during adulthood." In his article, Little explains that this process is a physiologic fact of life (maturational changes) which should be recognized as normal. He mentions that preventing this normal arch change with orthodontic treatment followed by retention only postpones the normal physiologic process. He emphasizes that permanent retention can block the process as long as the retainers are maintained but that once the retainers are removed, at whatever age, relapse to some degree will follow. He stresses that enlarging the lower arch during treatment only makes the case more prone to greater relapse and at a faster rate.

Patient C is an example of the treatment protocol recommended by the author to minimize post-retention relapse. Proclination of lower incisors was avoided by the extraction of four first bicuspids. This patient was successfully treated. However, he returned to the author's office 10 years post-retention with relapse of the alignment of his lower incisors, exemplifying the typical long-term post-retention lack of stability of lower incisor alignment.

The patient was a 15.4-year-old healthy male with a bilateral Class I malocclusion (Figs. 2.49, 2.50, and 2.51), with protrusive lips and a deficient chin (Fig. 2.52). His ANB angle was 2° (SNA 80°, SNB 78°), and his mandibular plane to SN was 30° (Fig. 2.53). His lower incisors were proclined relative to his mandibular plane (98°) and were 7 mm in front of the NB line. His maxillary incisors were 11 mm in front of the NA line and 108° to the SN line. He had a 3-mm anterior overjet and a 70 % overbite. His lower teeth were crowded with an arch length deficiency of 5 mm (Fig. 2.54), mainly on the right side resulting in the lower midline being shifted 2.5 mm toward the right. His maxillary arch had a minor rotation on the left central incisor (Fig. 2.55). He had suffered trauma on his maxillary left central and lateral incisors during a bicycle accident 1 year before and had required endodontic treatment. The left maxillary lateral incisor had a darker color than the rest of his teeth.

The patient and his parents were informed that extractions of 4 first premolars would be required to be able to reduce his dental and lip protrusion and also to level and align his teeth without proclining the incisors. They were also informed that full fixed appliances and a combination (cervical and occipital traction) headgear would also be required to improve the facial profile and to achieve an excellent occlusion and well-aligned teeth.

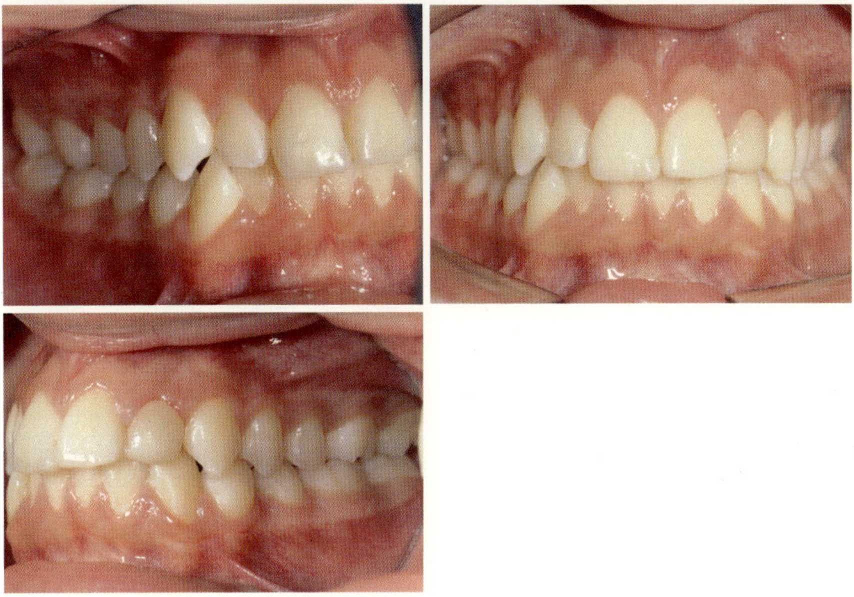

Figs. 2.49, 2.50, and 2.51 Pretreatment intraoral views with teeth in occlusion. Note Class I malocclusion with deep anterior overbite (70 %) and mandibular midline shifted 2.5 mm to the right side due to lower dental crowding mainly concentrated on the right side. Also note darkened color of the maxillary left lateral incisor. Both maxillary left incisors had required endodontic treatment due to a bicycle accident suffered 1 year previously

Treatment objectives were to level and align the teeth, to close the extraction spaces with maximum maxillary molar anchorage provided by a headgear, to maximize incisor retraction, and to reduce the lip protrusion. Mandibular growth was expected in this patient since he was a 15-year-old male with a father who was considerably taller. Thus, the HG was not only recommended to increase the anchorage but also to inhibit maxillary horizontal growth while mandibular growth proceeded, hopefully in a forward and downward direction. Both the patient and his parents accepted the treatment plan.

A combination headgear was given to the patient with instructions to wear it for 14 h per day. Full brackets were bonded to both dental arches, including second molars to increase anchorage, and a progression of arch wires were tied to all the brackets. En masse retraction of the incisors was carried out with edgewise wires. After 30 months of treatment, headgear wear was discontinued and the brackets were removed. A maxillary and a mandibular removable retainer were given to the patient with instructions to wear them nighttime for as long as he wished to have straight teeth. The patient was asked to have his left third molars extracted because the lower one was impacted. Also, internal bleaching of the two endodontically treated incisors was recommended because the crowns of these teeth appeared darker than the contralateral teeth.

The patient and his parents were very pleased with the results of the orthodontic treatment (Figs. 2.56, 2.57, 2.58, 2.59, 2.60, 2.61, and 2.62). The profile

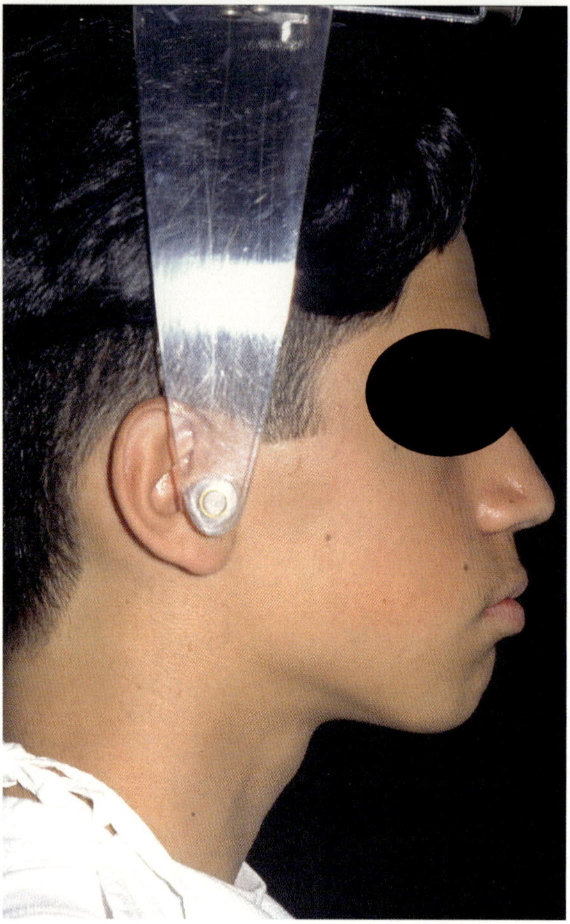

Fig. 2.52 Pretreatment facial profile view. Note protrusive lips and deficient chin

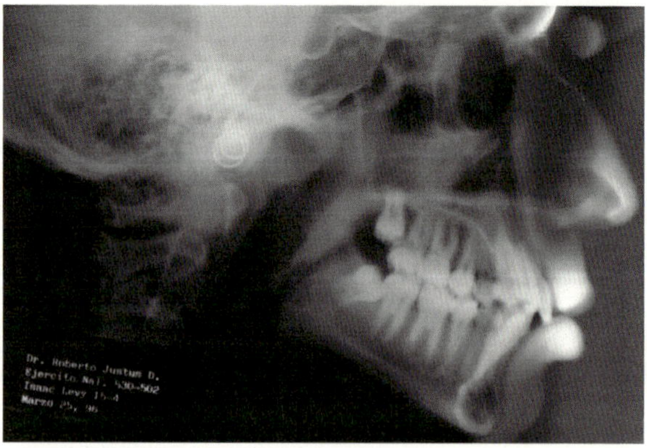

Fig. 2.53 Pretreatment cephalogram. Note proclined lower incisors (7 mm in front of the NB line and 98° relative to the mandibular plane) and proclined maxillary incisors (11 mm in front of the NA line and 108° relative to the SN line)

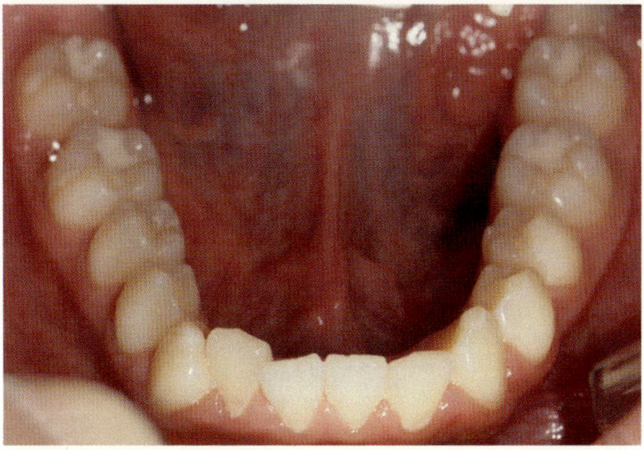

Fig. 2.54 Pretreatment intraoral mandibular occlusal view. Note 5-mm arch length deficiency

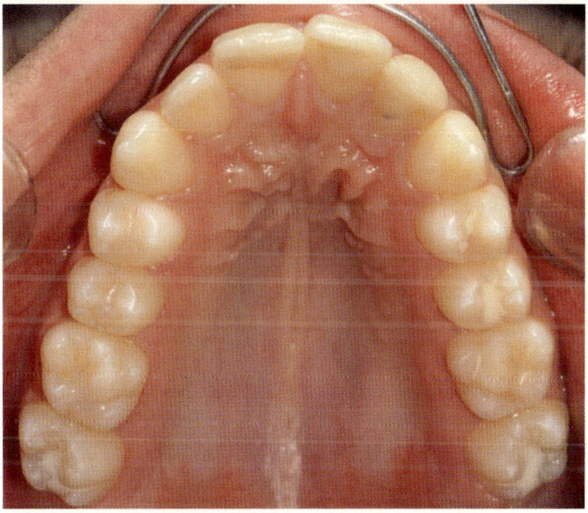

Fig. 2.55 Pretreatment intraoral maxillary occlusal view. Note minimum dental crowding with maxillary left central incisor rotated mesio-labially

improvement was dramatic when one compares the pre- and the posttreatment facial photographs (Figs. 2.52 and 2.60) because the chin projection increased and lip protrusion decreased. The cranial base lateral headfilm superimposition tracing (Fig. 2.63) demonstrates excellent mandibular growth, in a forward and downward direction, which helped to project forward his originally deficient chin. The tracing also demonstrates excellent headgear cooperation because the maxilla was inhibited from growing forward making it easy to correct the anterior overjet and overbite taking advantage of the excellent mandibular growth. Both maxillary (Fig. 2.64) and mandibular superimpositions (Fig. 2.65) demonstrate excellent incisor retraction which allowed the lips to have a normal posture (not protrusive). His lower incisors, which were originally proclined relative to his mandibular plane at 98°, are now at 93°. These incisors were 7 mm in front of the NB line and are now at 3 mm; his maxillary incisors changed from being 11 mm to 3 mm in front of the NA line and from 108° to 82° with respect to the SN line.

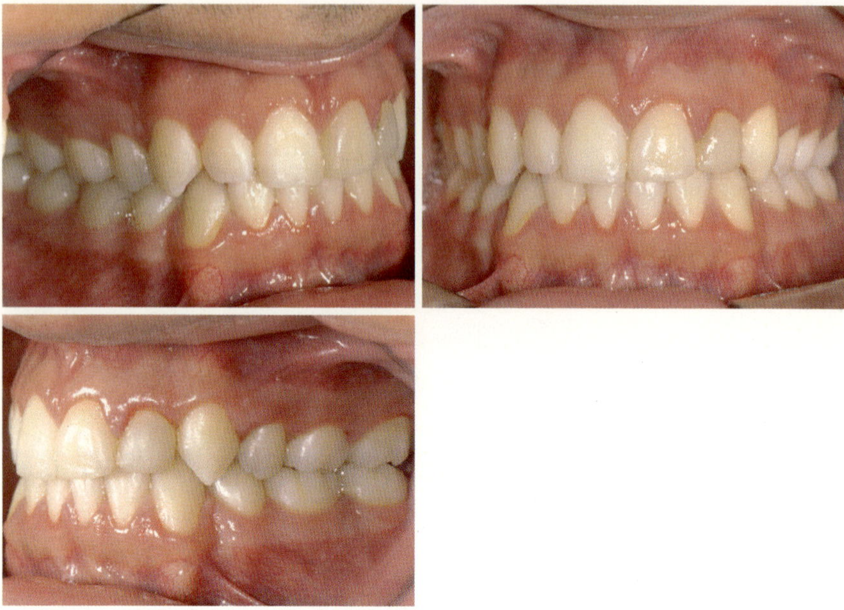

Figs. 2.56, 2.57, and 2.58 Posttreatment intraoral views with teeth in occlusion. Note good occlusion and dental midline coincidence. Also note that maxillary left incisors appear darker in color; internal bleaching of these two teeth was recommended

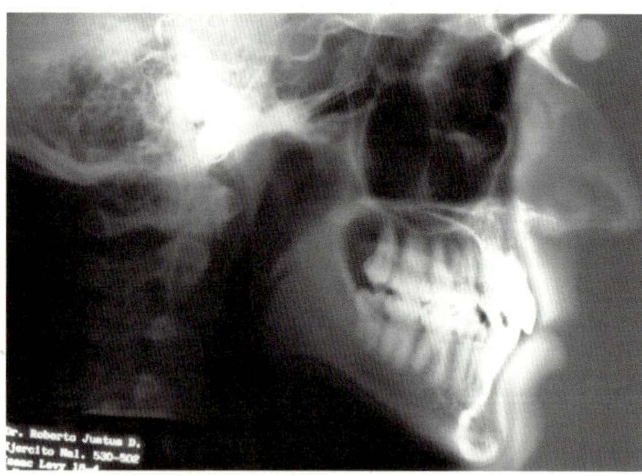

Fig. 2.59 Posttreatment cephalogram. Note upright lower incisors (3 mm in front of the NB line and 93° relative to the mandibular plane). Also note upright maxillary incisors (3 mm in front of the NA line and 83° relative to the SN line)

Posttreatment records were taken, and the patient was instructed to return for annual retainer checkups and also to evaluate the eruption of his right third molars. The patient however did not return for 14 years. When he showed up, the author was very happy to see that he had maintained his pleasing profile (Fig. 2.66) and that the mandibular right third molar had erupted in a correct alignment (Fig. 2.67) and was in a good occlusion (Fig. 2.68), but he exhibited posttreatment relapse of the lower incisor alignment (Fig. 2.67) because he had discontinued using his retainers. He

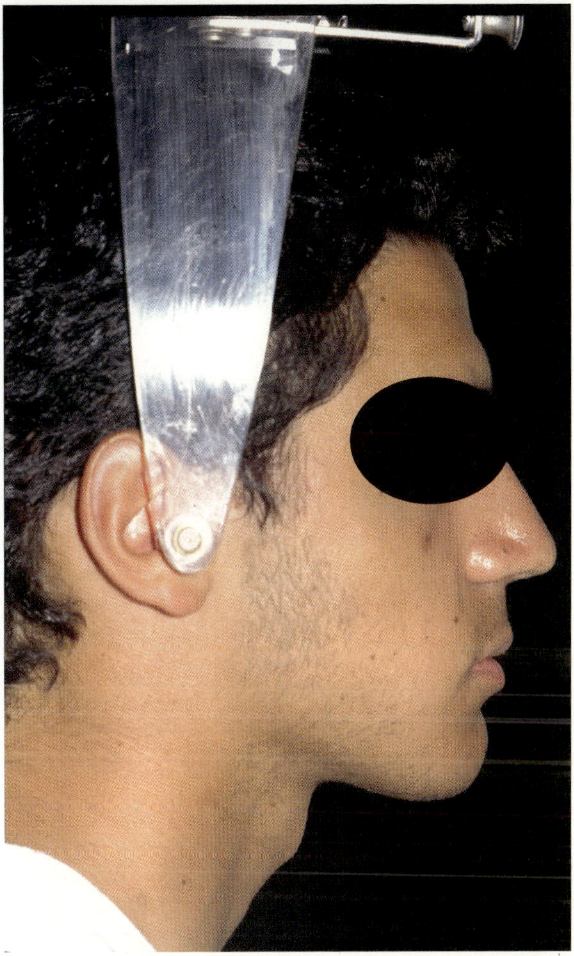

Fig. 2.60 Posttreatment facial profile view. Note a pleasing profile due to increased chin projection and decreased lip protrusion

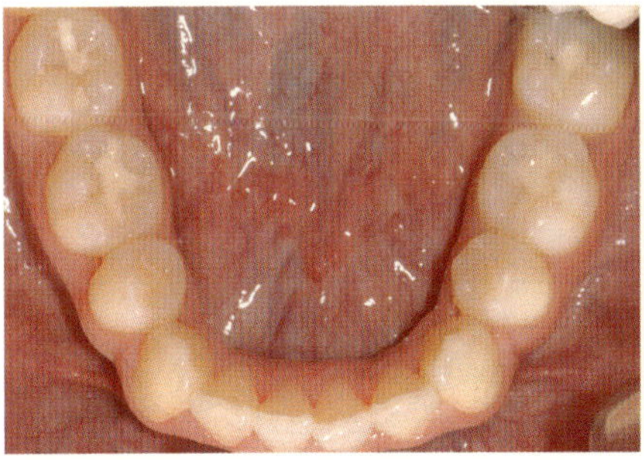

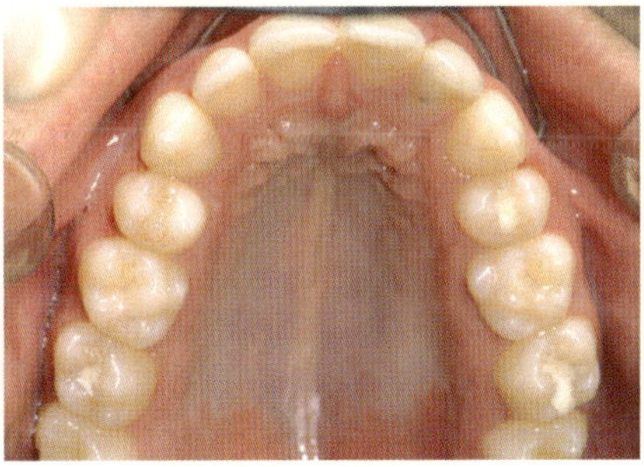

Figs. 2.61 and 2.62 Posttreatment intraoral occlusal mandibular and maxillary views. Note acceptable dental alignment

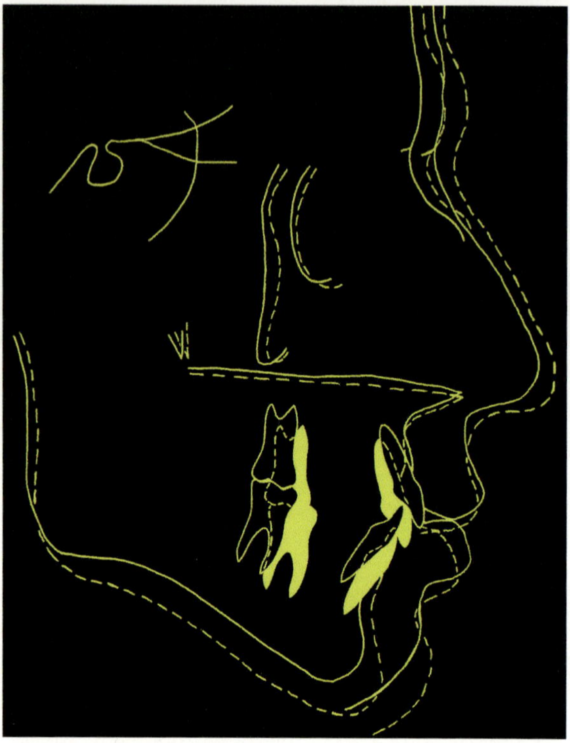

Fig. 2.63 Cranial base superimposition of cephalogram tracings, ages 15.4 and 18.4. Note excellent mandibular growth while maxillary anterior growth in a forward direction was inhibited by good headgear use

confessed to having used them for only 4 years after having finished his orthodontic treatment. The patient asked to be retreated not only because the lower incisors had alignment relapse but also because the left first and second molars were in lingual crossbite (Figs. 2.69 and 2.70). The patient was retreated successfully (Figs. 2.71, 2.72, 2.73, and 2.74) with full fixed appliances and given a maxillary wraparound and a mandibular removable retainer (Fig. 2.75).

In this case, extraction treatment greatly improved this patient's profile and resolved his dental crowding, but in spite of having avoided incisor proclination, crowding increased post-retention. Evidence shows that this alignment relapse would have been greater had non-extraction treatment been prescribed for this patient.

2.5 Deficient Chin Projection Appearance and Lip Incompetence Associated with Lower Incisor Proclination

Facial esthetics could be compromised in some patients if lower incisors are moved labially because as the teeth procline, the lips also move forward, while the chin stays back. Thus, an increase in lip protrusion is associated with the appearance of

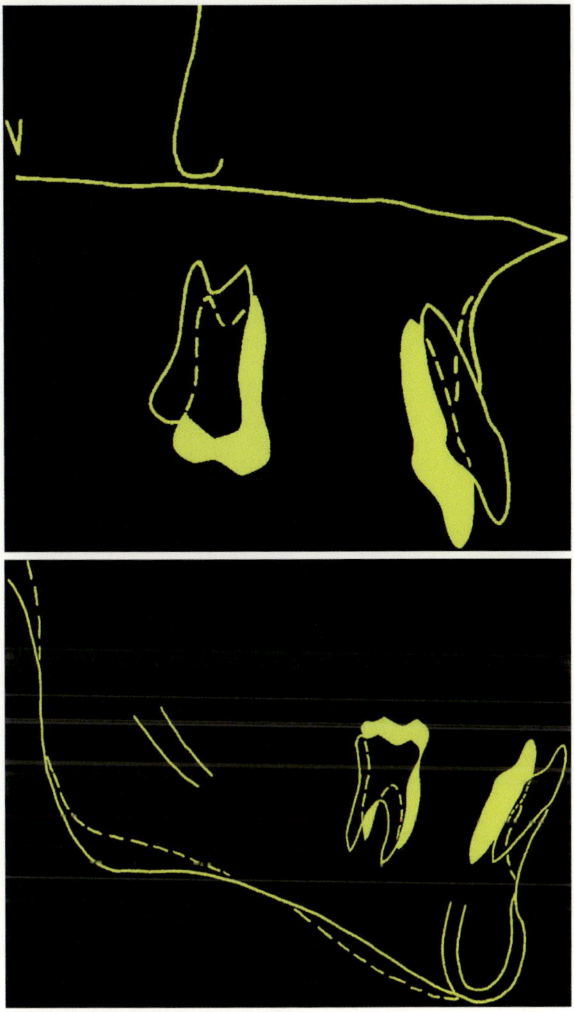

Figs. 2.64 and 2.65 Maxillary and mandibular cephalometric superimpositions of tracings, ages 15.4 and 18.4. Note excellent incisor retraction which helped to normalize the original double lip protrusion and also the relationship between soft tissue pogonion and inferior labrale

a decreased chin projection and a diminished labiomental sulcus. Incisor proclination may certainly compromise facial esthetics in some patients.

Patient B is an example of the negative impact that non-extraction orthodontic treatment has on both lip protrusion and the lack of chin projection in patients who have arch length deficiency. In patient B, the incisors were proclined during orthodontic treatment. Patient C, on the other hand, is an example of the positive impact that four first bicuspid extraction orthodontic treatment had on the teeth, on the lips, and on the chin projection, because the incisors were retracted.

The posttreatment anteroposterior position of the incisors determines the drape of the lips and is therefore very often at the heart of orthodontic treatment planning [28–31]. For most clinicians, the treatment plan revolves around the eventual position of the anterior teeth in the face and the establishment of an excellent occlusion.

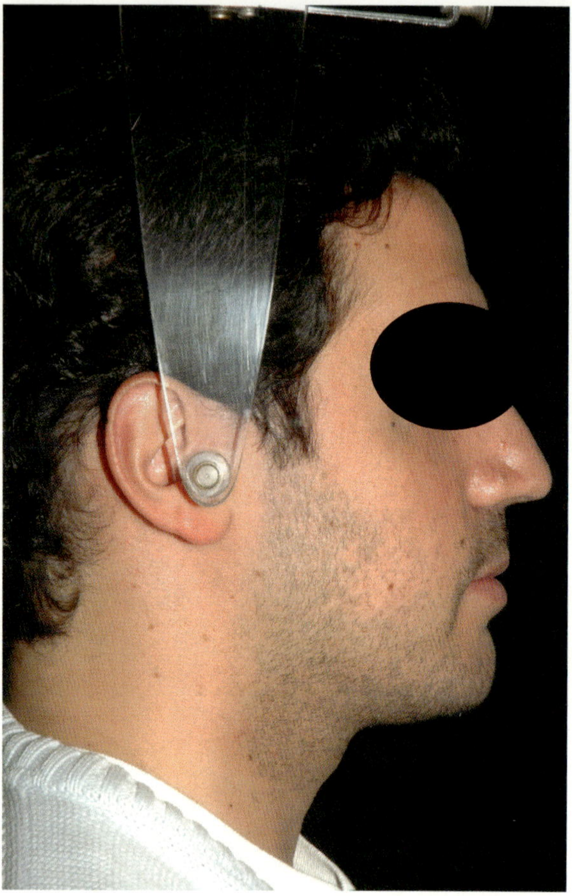

Fig. 2.66 Ten-year post-retention facial profile view, age 32.2. Note good facial balance was maintained

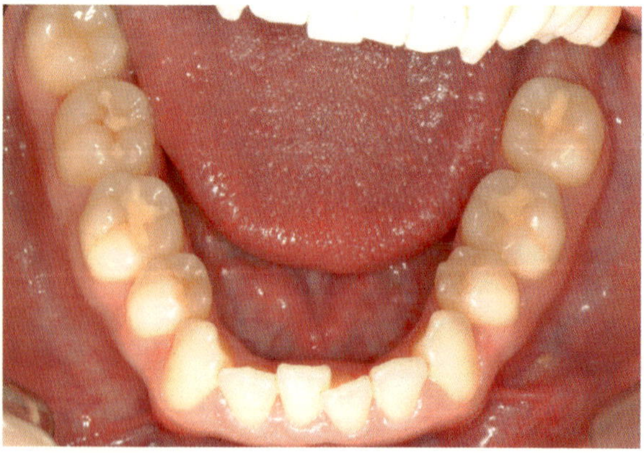

Fig. 2.67 Ten-year post-retention mandibular occlusal view. Note incisor irregularity

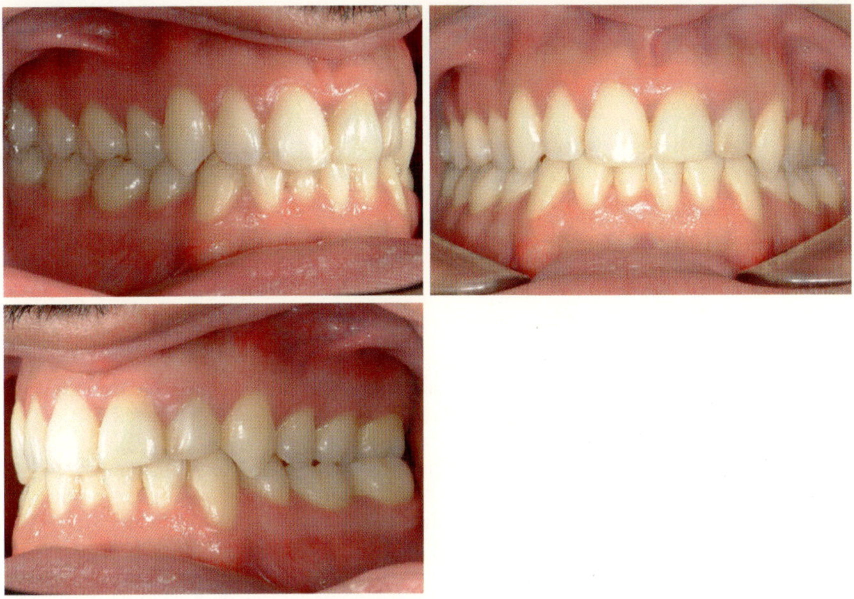

Figs. 2.68, 2.69, and 2.70 Ten-year post-retention intraoral views with teeth in occlusion. Note third molars on the right side are in good occlusion; however, maxillary left first and second molars are in lingual crossbite. Additionally, the two maxillary left incisors still have a darker color relative to the rest of the teeth. Endodontic re-treatment of these two teeth was recommended

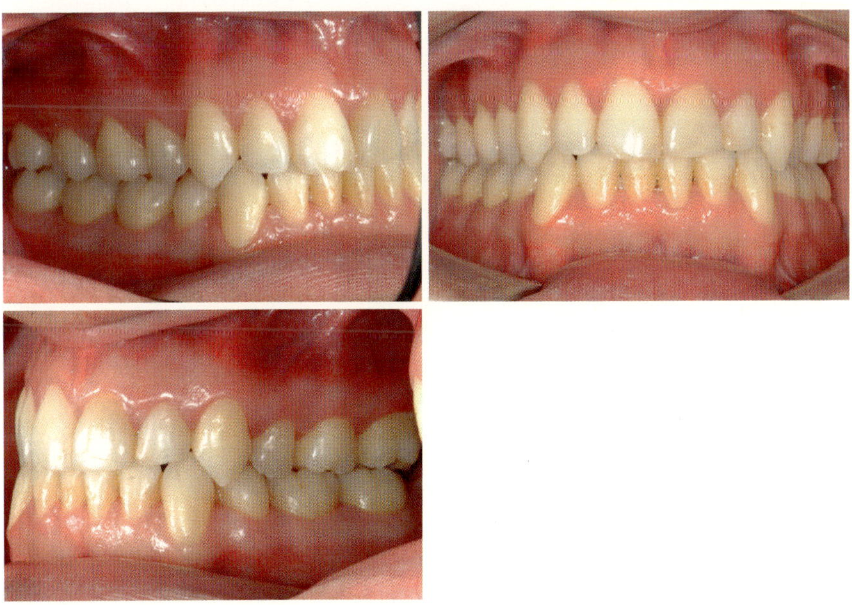

Figs. 2.71, 2.72, and 2.73 Post-re-treatment intraoral views with teeth in occlusion, age 32.10. Note good occlusion and improvement in the color of the two maxillary left incisors due to endodontic re-treatment and internal bleaching

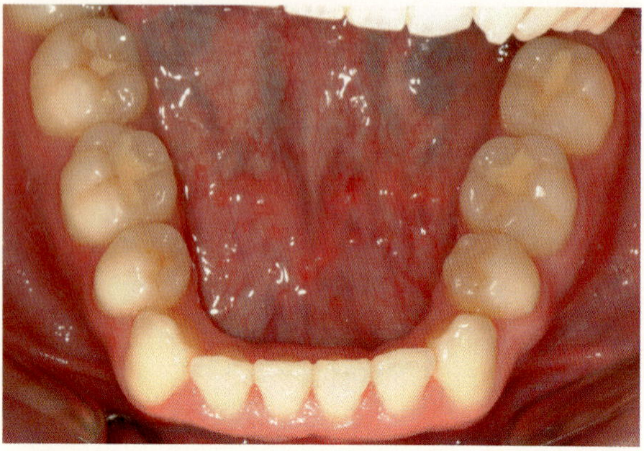

Fig. 2.74 Post-re-treatment intraoral mandibular occlusal view, age 32.10. Note good dental alignment

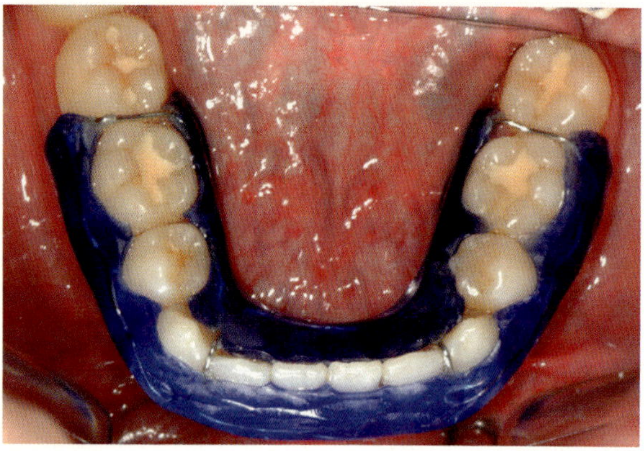

Fig. 2.75 Post-re-treatment intraoral mandibular occlusal view with removable retainer, age 32.10. Note labial and lingual acrylic covering all teeth from first molar to first molar to guarantee perfect alignment. This removable retainer is to be worn nightly as long as patient wishes to have perfectly aligned teeth

It has often been claimed that extraction treatment has a "flattening" effect on the facial profile. In patients who exhibit dental crowding in their lower arch, but in whom no lip retraction is required because of a good pretreatment profile, the author recommends extracting the upper first bicuspids and lower second bicuspids. By using this extraction pattern, the facial profile is better protected from flattening.

It is widely accepted that there is a strong relation between root surface area and anchorage and that the choice of teeth extracted therefore has a direct effect on the magnitude of anterior segment retraction. This has led to the concept of differential extractions. Proffit and Fields [28] state that ".....all other things being equal, the amount of incisor retraction will be less, the further posteriorly in the arch an extraction is located" and that "..... even with second premolar extraction, some retraction of the lower incisors may occur, but most of the space closure will be by mesial movement of the lower molars."

Evidence of less incisor retraction with the extraction of lower second bicuspids than with extraction of first bicuspids is given by many authors [28–30]. Steyn et al. [31] found that the lower incisors were retracted slightly more in a group of patients in whom four first premolars were extracted than in two groups in which lower second bicuspids were extracted (one group had four second bicuspids extracted while the other group had upper first bicuspids and lower second bicuspids extracted). Shearn et al. [29] found that increased lower incisor retraction occurred in lower first premolar extraction than in lower second premolar extraction cases. Luppanapornlap and Johnston [30] reported that lower first premolar extractions had on average a 3-mm retrusive effect on lower incisors, compared with a 2-mm retrusive effect for lower second premolar extractions. Similar mean findings were found by both Steyn et al. and Shearn et al. The conclusion from these three studies is that there is an indication for the extraction of second bicuspids when the objective is to minimize facial flattening. This extraction pattern maximizes mesial movement of the lower molars but still provides sufficient space to align crowded teeth while simultaneously protecting the facial profile from flattening. Thus, lower incisor retraction is minimized which in turn also minimizes maxillary incisor retraction maintaining thereby a better lip support.

If incisor crowding is minimal (less than 4-mm arch length discrepancy) in a patient with a pleasing profile, extraction therapy might not be indicated. However, in order to avoid proclining the incisors during the orthodontic alignment of such patients, interproximal reduction (stripping) might be indicated.

Contemporary extraction guidelines are given in the textbook *Contemporary Orthodontics* [5]. For the benefit of the reader, the following is a brief summary. When the prominence of the incisors creates excessive lip separation at rest, so the patient must strain to bring the lips together, the teeth are too protrusive and retracting the incisors improves facial appearance. An individual with thick, full lips looks good with incisor prominence that would not be acceptable in someone with thin, tight lips. The size of the nose and chin has a profound effect on relative lip prominence. For a patient with a large nose and/or a large chin, if the choices are to treat without extraction and move the incisors forward, or extract and retract the incisors at least somewhat, moving the incisors forward is better, provided it does not diminish the labiomental sulcus too much. Lack of a well-defined labiomental sulcus, which usually is related to lipstrain in gaining lip seal, can be due either to increased lower face height or protrusion of the teeth, and this also can be taken as evidence that the incisors are too prominent. A concave profile with thinning of the lips, so that there is little vermilion border, is an unesthetic trait. In a patient with thin lips, proclining the incisors tends to create fuller lips with more vermilion display, and this is likely to be perceived as more attractive. Since the face tends to flatten with age and the lips become less full with aging, retracting teeth in a patient with thin lips can prematurely age the face. The upper lip should be slightly forward from its base at soft tissue point A. For best esthetics, the lower lip should be at least as prominent as the chin.

The abovementioned extraction guidelines are only a few that the clinician must take into account before deciding whether to extract or not in a particular patient. The author recommends that all the above considerations be taken into account, including the arch length discrepancy, in order to make a wise decision whether to extract in any particular patient.

The following patient report is a good example of how the author was able to align crowded teeth without proclining the incisors, by extracting maxillary first

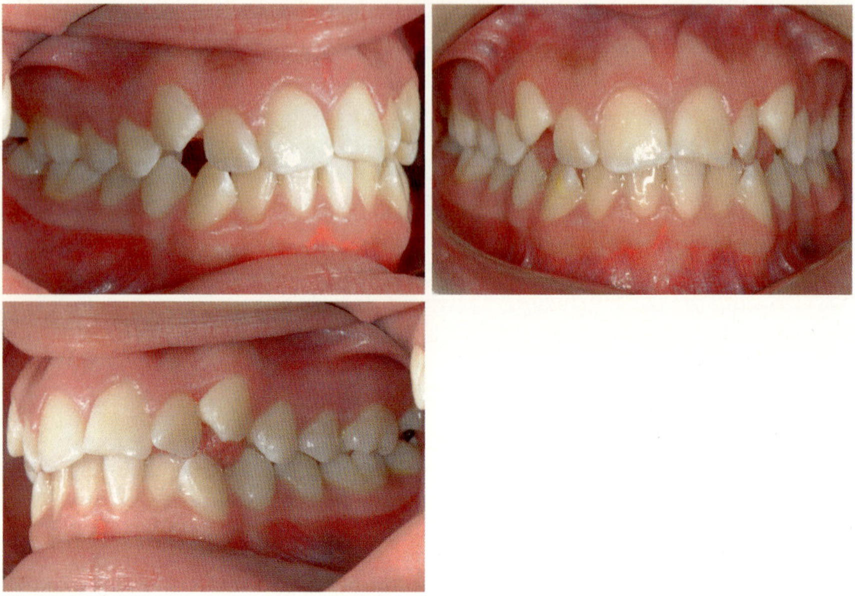

Figs. 2.76, 2.77, and 2.78 Pretreatment intraoral views with teeth in occlusion. Note Class I malocclusion with maxillary and mandibular dental crowding. Maxillary left central incisor had suffered trauma in a swimming pool accident and had fractured its incisal border

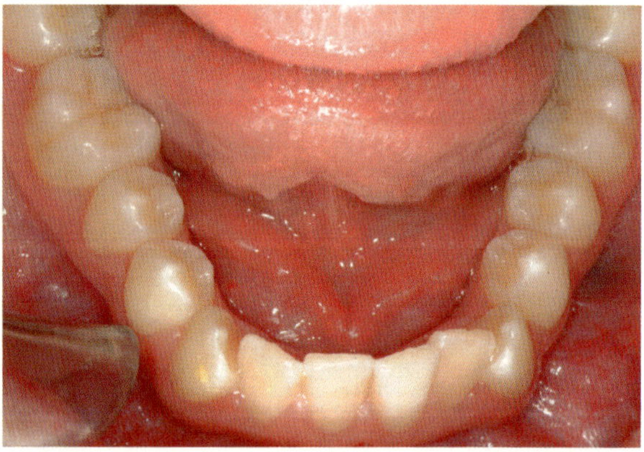

Fig. 2.79 Pretreatment intraoral mandibular occlusal view. Note 5-mm arch length deficiency

bicuspids and mandibular second bicuspids, while simultaneously protecting the profile from flattening, by not over-retracting the incisors.

Patient D was a 12.1-year-old healthy girl who had a bilateral Class I malocclusion with crowding (Figs. 2.76, 2.77, 2.78, 2.79, and 2.80). She had a perfectly positioned upper lip in profile view, a deficient chin with no mentolabial sulcus, and a dorsal nasal hump (Fig. 2.81). Skeletally, she was Class II (Fig. 2.82) with an ANB angle of 6° (SNA 79°, SNB 73°), mainly due to a retrusive mandible. Her mandibular plane to the SN line was 47°. Her lower incisors were retroclined relative to her

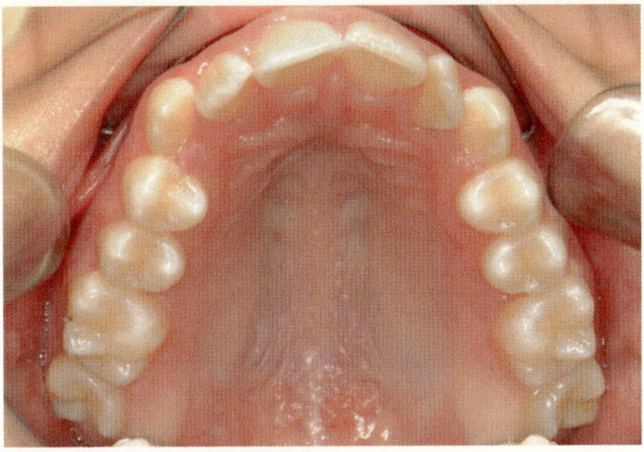

Fig. 2.80 Pretreatment intraoral maxillary occlusal view. Note 5-mm arch length deficiency and fractured incisal border of the left central incisor

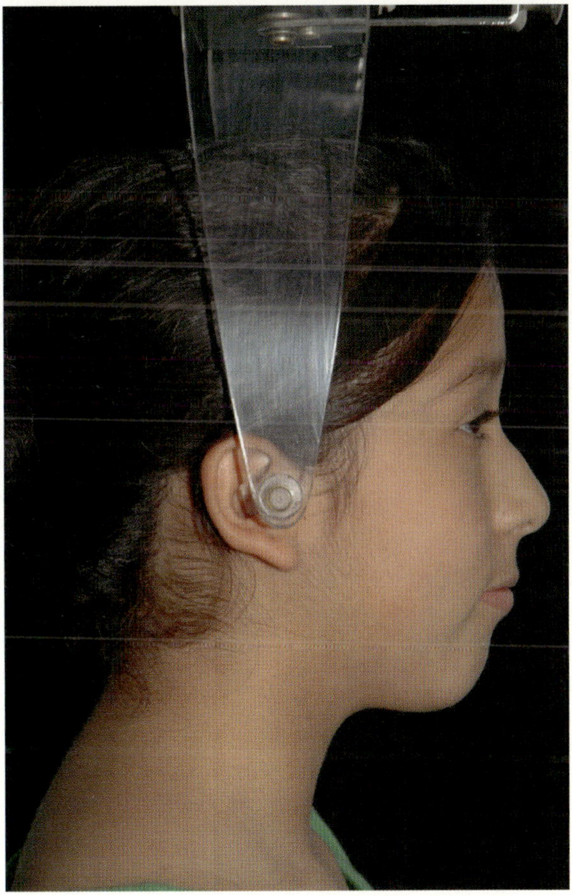

Fig. 2.81 Pretreatment facial profile view. Note Class II facial profile with a pleasing upper lip but an elongated lower lip associated with a high mandibular plane angle (47° to SN). Also note a nasal hump and a deficient chin without a well-defined labiomental sulcus

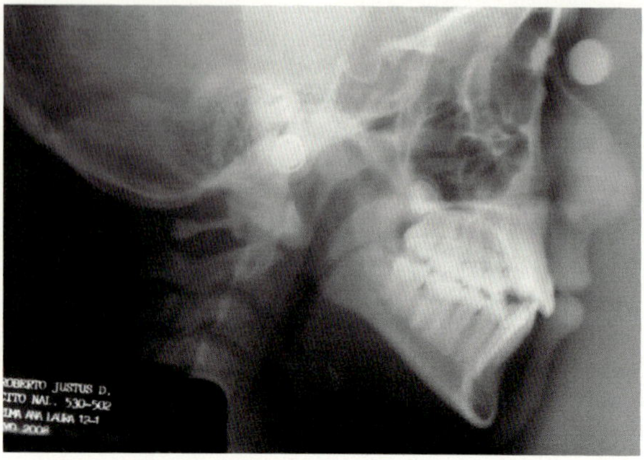

Fig. 2.82 Pretreatment cephalogram. Note proclined lower incisors (8.5 mm in front of the NB line) but retroclined at 82° relative to the mandibular plane, probably due to a high mandibular plane of 47°. The maxillary incisors were normally positioned (2 mm in front of the NA line and 98° relative to the SN line). Also note an ANB angle of 6°

mandibular plane (82°) but were proclined 8.5 mm in front of the NB line, and her maxillary incisors were 2 mm in front of the NA line and 98° to the SN line. She had a 3-mm anterior overjet and a 70 % overbite. Both maxillary and mandibular dentitions were crowded with an arch length deficiency of 5 mm (Figs. 2.79 and 2.80). She had suffered a swimming pool accident with trauma to her maxillary left central incisor which fractured the incisal border of this tooth (Fig. 2.77). Her menarche had occurred only 6 months before so some growth was still expected.

The patient and her parents were informed that extractions were necessary to be able to level and align her teeth without proclining incisors and that extraction of second mandibular premolars and maxillary first premolars would protect her profile from flattening. They were also informed that full fixed appliances and a combination (cervical and occipital traction) headgear would also be required, the latter to improve her chin projection through mandibular growth while her maxillary forward growth was being restrained. Also explained was the fact that some lower incisor retraction would help give the chin the appearance of being more forward and also improve its definition through the creation of a labiomental sulcus. Plastic surgery was recommended to eliminate her dorsal nasal hump.

Treatment objectives were to level and align the teeth, to close the extraction spaces with minimum anchorage, to maintain the upper lip position, and to increase chin prominence. As mentioned before, some mandibular growth was expected in this patient since she had had her menarche 6 months previously and some residual growth was anticipated. The headgear was recommended to inhibit maxillary horizontal growth while mandibular growth proceeded, hopefully in a forward and downward direction so the chin definition and prominence would improve. Both the patient and her parents accepted the treatment plan.

A combination headgear was given to the patient with instructions to wear it for 14 h per day. The maxillary first bicuspids and the mandibular second bicuspids were extracted. Full brackets were then bonded to both dental arches, including second molars, and a progression of arch wires were tied to all the brackets. En masse extraction space closure was carried out with edgewise wires, applying labial crown torque on the incisors to maximize mesial molar movement. Ten months after

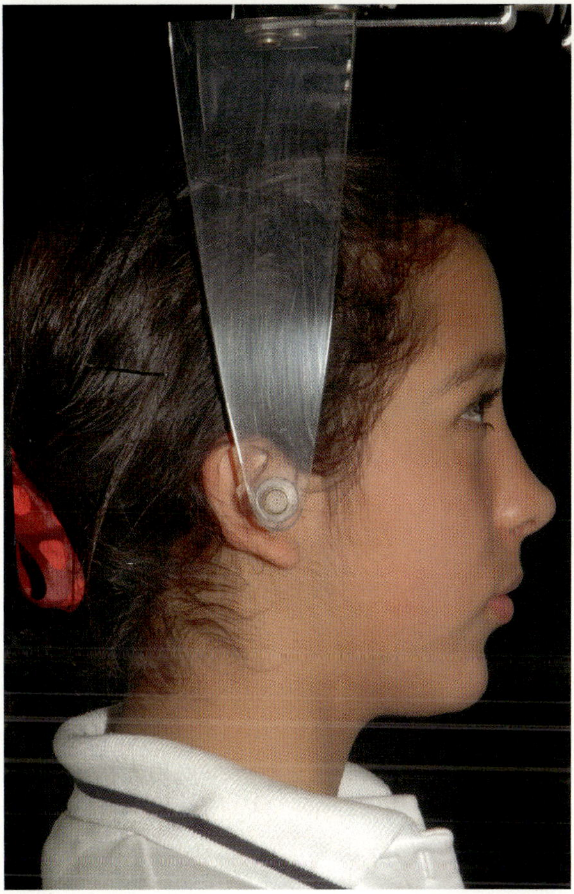

Fig. 2.83 Thirteen-month progress facial profile view, after plastic surgery to eliminate the nasal hump. Note that the upper lip was not retracted in spite of having closed extraction spaces because lower second and upper first bicuspids were extracted. Space closure of the extraction spaces improved the chin projection appearance and gave a better definition of the mentolabial sulcus. Class II facial profile still remains

bracket placement, the patient underwent nasal rhinoplasty to remove her dorsal nasal hump (Fig. 2.83). After 30 months of treatment, headgear wear was discontinued, and the brackets were removed. Maxillary and mandibular removable retainers were given to the patient with instructions to wear them nighttime for as long as she wished to have straight teeth. Posttreatment records were taken and instructions were given to the patient to return annually for retainer checkups and to observe whether the third molars would erupt in a correct position.

The patient and her parents were very pleased with the treatment results (Figs. 2.84, 2.85, 2.86, 2.87, and 2.88). The profile improvement was dramatic when one compares the pre- and the posttreatment facial profile photographs (Figs. 2.81 and 2.89) and the pre- and post-cephalograms (Figs. 2.82 and 2.90) because the chin projection increased, a labiomental sulcus was created, and the lower lip protrusion decreased. The cranial base lateral headfilm superimposition tracing (Fig. 2.91) demonstrates some mandibular growth had indeed occurred. This growth combined with the lower incisor retraction helped to give the chin a more prominent appearance and the creation of a well-defined labiomental sulcus. The superimposition

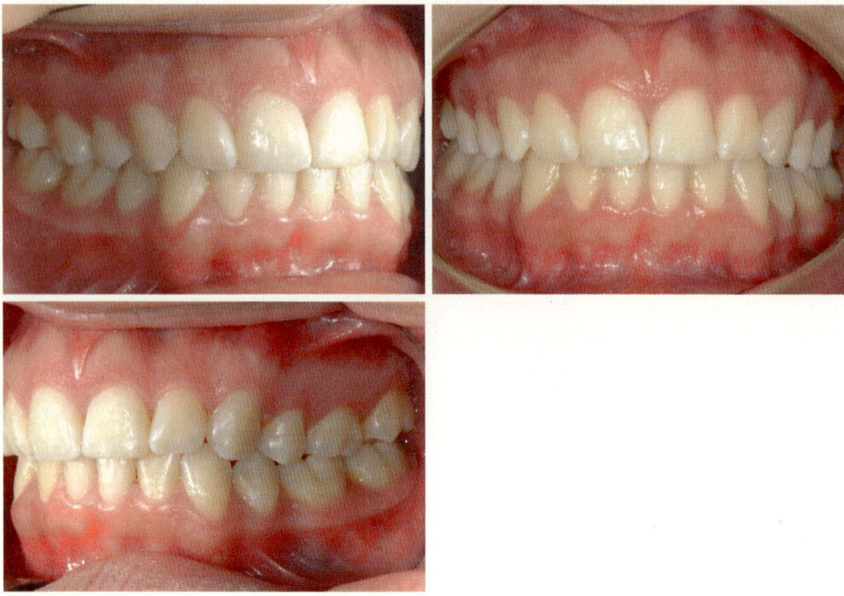

Figs. 2.84, 2.85, and 2.86 Posttreatment intraoral views with teeth in occlusion, age 16.6. Note good occlusion and dental midline coincidence

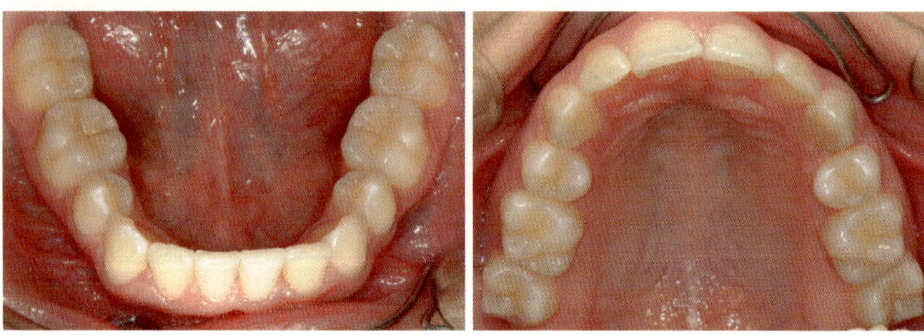

Figs. 2.87 and 2.88 Posttreatment intraoral occlusal mandibular and maxillary views. Note acceptable dental alignment

also demonstrates excellent headgear cooperation because the maxilla was inhibited from growing forward making it easier to correct the anterior overjet and overbite by taking advantage of the mandibular growth that took place. Both maxillary (Fig. 2.92) and mandibular superimpositions (Fig. 2.93) demonstrate sufficient incisor retraction which allowed the lips to have a normal posture. Her lower incisors, which were originally proclined relative to the NB line at 8.5 mm, are now at 7 mm, compensating for a retrusive mandible. These incisors were initially at 82° relative to the mandibular plane and are now 90°. Her maxillary incisors changed from being 2 mm in front of the NA line to 0 mm and from 97° to 88° with respect

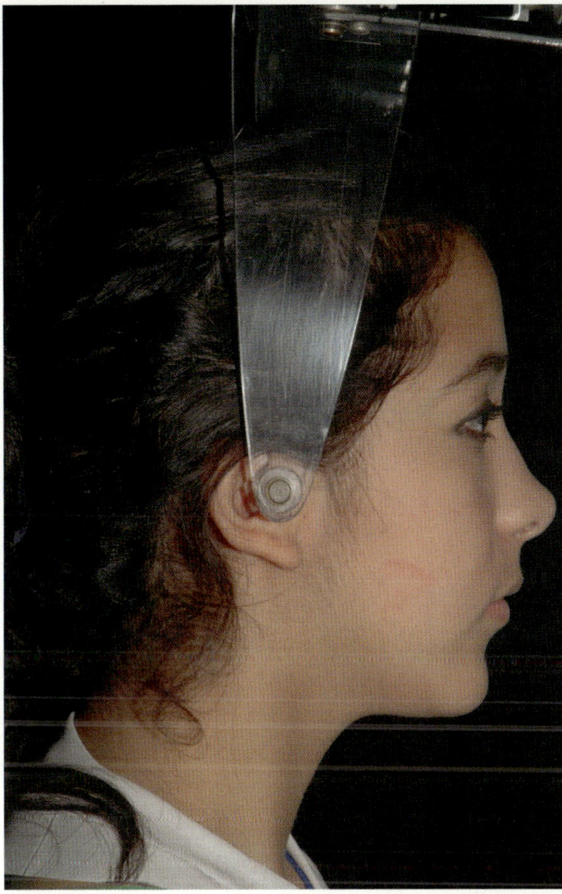

Fig. 2.89 Posttreatment facial profile view. Note a pleasing profile due to increased chin projection and decreased lip protrusion. Upper lip was protected from retraction due to the extraction of lower second and upper first bicuspids. Class II facial profile still remains

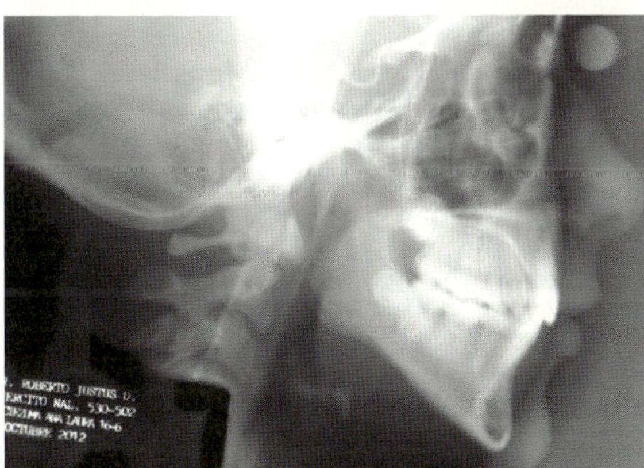

Fig. 2.90 Posttreatment cephalogram. Note upright lower incisors (7 mm in front of the NB line and 90° relative to the mandibular plane). Also note upright maxillary incisors (0 mm with respect to the NA line and 88° relative to the SN line). The ANB of 6° remained the same; thus, dental compensations for the skeletal imbalance were necessary

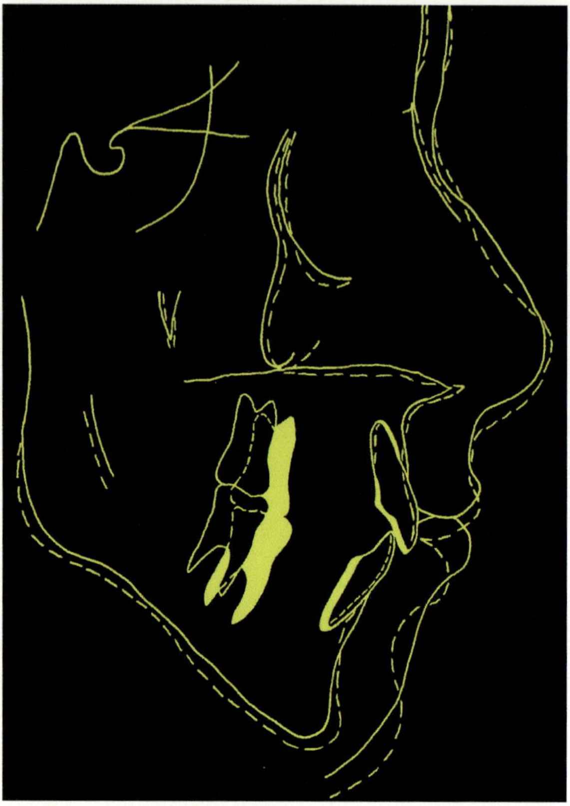

Fig. 2.91 Cranial base superimposition of cephalogram tracings, ages 12.1 and 16.6. Note some mandibular growth and bone deposition at pogonion. Also note change in nasal form due to plastic surgery

to the SN line. These are the dental compensations that were necessary to achieve a good occlusion taking into account the Class II skeletal pattern the patient had with an ANB angle of 6°.

In cases such as that of patient D, in which extractions are required to alleviate crowding but in whom flattening the upper lip is contraindicated, differential premolar extraction is indeed an optimal extraction pattern which does not compromise facial esthetics.

2.6 Concluding Remarks

It is the author's hope that this second chapter will create awareness among clinicians that mandibular arch expansion (arch development) to alleviate dental crowding should generally be avoided. The initial facial profile, the degree of crowding, and the gingival type should guide the orthodontist in establishing his or her treatment plan. Finally, if extraction therapy is indicated, the clinician has many choices of different extraction patterns to achieve the best facial harmony.

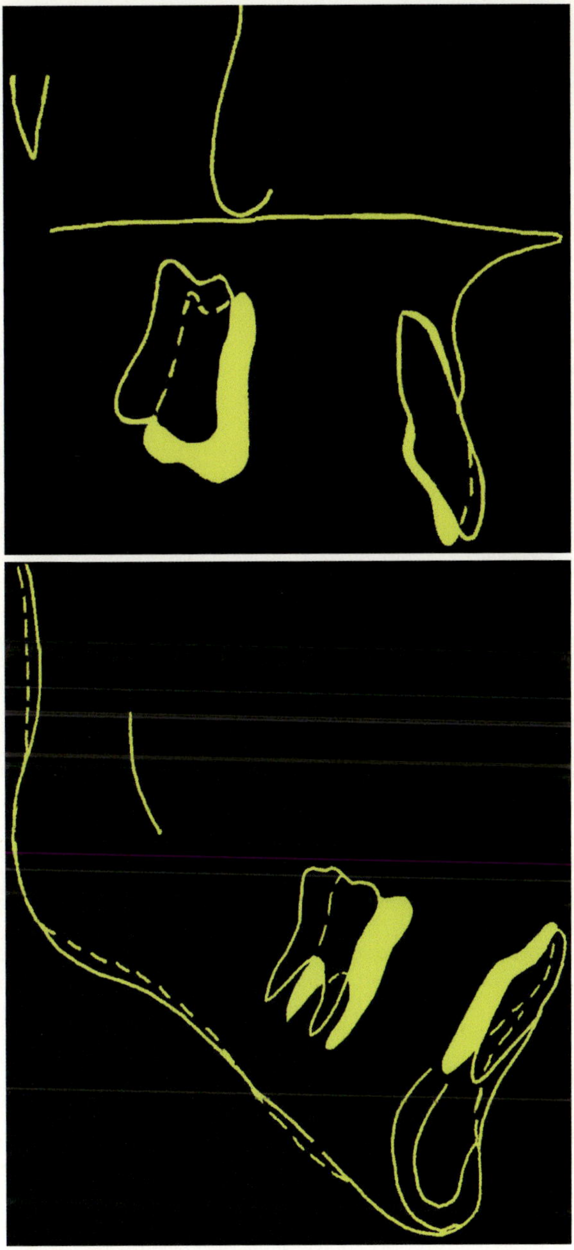

Figs. 2.92 and 2.93 Maxillary and mandibular cephalometric superimpositions of tracings, ages 12.1 and 16.6. Note more mesial movement of maxillary and mandibular molars which helped to minimize the retraction of incisors. This was due to having extracted lower second and upper first bicuspids. Upper incisors were uprighted to compensate for the skeletal Class II with an ANB of 6° which did not improve during treatment

References

1. Slutzkey S, Levin L. Gingival recession in young adults: occurrence, severity, and relationship to past orthodontic treatment and oral piercing. Am J Orthod Dentofacial Orthop. 2008;134:652–6.
2. Bollen AM, Cunha CJ, Bakko DW, et al. Effects of orthodontic therapy on periodontal health: a systematic review of controlled evidence. J Am Dent Assoc. 2008;139:413–22.
3. Wennström JL. Mucogingival considerations in orthodontic treatment. Semin Orthod. 1996;2:46–54.
4. Bowman SJ. Altering the extraction decision with mini-screws. J Clin Orthod. 2011;10:42–9.
5. Proffit WR, Fields HW, Sarver DM. Contemporary orthodontics. 4th ed. Saint Louis: Mosby, Inc. USA; 2007. p. 279–83.
6. Ochseinbein C, Ross S. A reevaluation of osseous surgery. Dent Clin North Am. 1969;13: 87–102.
7. Seibert JL, Lindhe J. Esthetics and periodontal therapy. In: Lindhe J, editor. Textbook of clinical periodontology. 2nd ed. Copenhagen: Munksgaard; 1989. p. 477–514.
8. Kao RT, Fagan MC, Conte GJ. Thick vs. thin gingival biotypes: a key determinant in treatment planning for dental implants. CDA J. 2008;36:193–8.
9. Cook DR, Mealey BL, Verrett RG, et al. Relationship between clinical periodontal biotype and labial plate thickness: an in vivo study. Int J Periodontics Restorative Dent. 2011;31:345–54.
10. Foushee DG, Moriarty JD, Simpson DM. Effects of mandibular orthognathic treatment on mucogingival tissues. J Periodontol. 1985;56:727–33.
11. Zachrisson BU. Orthodontics and periodontics. In: Lindhe J, Karring T, Lang NP, editors. Clinical periodontology and implant dentistry. 3rd ed. Copenhagen: Munksgaard; 1997. p. 741–93.
12. Claffey N, Shanley D. Relationship of gingival thickness and bleeding to loss of probing attachment in shallow sites following non surgical periodontal therapy. J Clin Periodontol. 1986;13:654–7.
13. De Rouck T, Eghbali R, Collys K, et al. The gingival biotype revisited: transparency of the periodontal probe through the gingival margin as a method to discriminate thin from thick gingiva. J Clin Peridontol. 2009;36:428–33.
14. Olsson M, Lindhe J. Periodontal characteristics in individuals with varying form of the upper central incisors. J Clin Periodontol. 1991;18:78–82.
15. Wennström JL, Lindhe J, Sinclair F, et al. Some periodontal tissue reaction to orthodontic tooth movement in monkeys. J Clin Periodontol. 1987;14:121–9.
16. Wennström JL. Lack of association between width of attached gingiva and development of gingival recession. A 5 year longitudinal study. J Clin Periodontol. 1987;14:181–4.
17. Proffit WR, Phillips C, Dann C, et al. Stability after surgical-orthodontic correction of skeletal Class III malocclusion. I. Mandibular setback. Int J Adult Orthodon Orthognath Surg. 1991;6:7–18.
18. Justus R. Finalizaci6n en Ortodoncia. In: Interlandi S, editor. Ortodoncia–Bases para la Iniciaci6n. Sao Paulo: Editorial Artes Médicas; 2002. p. 533–46.
19. Little RM, Wallen T, Riedel RA, et al. Stability and relapse of mandibular anterior alignment—first premolar extraction cases treated by traditional edgewise orthodontics. Am J Orthod. 1981;80:349–65.
20. Little RM, Riedel RA, Årtun J. An evaluation of changes in mandibular anterior alignment from 10 to 20 years post-retention. Am J Orthod Dentofacial Orthop. 1988;93:423–8.
21. Little RM, Riedel RA, Engst ED. Serial extraction of first premolars – postretention evaluation of stability and relapse. Angle Orthod. 1990;60:255–62.
22. McReynolds DC, Little RM. Mandibular second premolar extraction – postretention evaluation of stability and relapse. Angle Orthod. 1991;61:133–44.
23. Riedel RA, Little RM, Bui TD. Mandibular incisor extraction—postretention evaluation of stability and relapse. Angle Orthod. 1992;62:103–16.

24. Little RM, Riedel RA. Postretention evaluation of stability and relapse—mandibular arches with generalized spacing. Am J Orthod Dentofacial Orthop. 1989;95:37–41.
25. Little RM, Riedel RA, Stein A. Mandibular arch length increase during the mixed dentition: postretention evaluation of stability and relapse. Am J Orthod Dentofacial Orthop. 1990;97:393–404.
26. Sinclair PM. Clinical implications of the University of Washington post-retention studies. Interview with Dr. RM Little. J Clin Orthod. 2009;43:645–51.
27. Al Yami EA, Kuijpers-Jagtman A, van't Hof MA. Stability of orthodontic treatment outcome: follow-up until 10 years post-retention. Am J Orthod Dentofacial Orthop. 1999;115:300–4.
28. Steyn CL, du Preez RJ, Harris AMP. Differential premolar extraction. Am J Orthod Dentofacial Orthop. 1997;112:480–6.
29. Proffit WR, Fields HW. Contemporary orthodontics. 2nd ed. Saint Louis: Mosby, Inc.; 1993.
30. Shearn BN, Woods MG. An occlusal and cephalometric analysis of lower 1st and 2nd premolar extraction effects. Am J Orthod Dentofacial Orthop. 2000;117:351–61.
31. Luppanapornlap S, Johnston L. The effect of premolar extraction: a long-term comparison of outcomes in "clear-cut" extraction and nonextraction Class II patients. Angle Orthod. 1993;63:257–72.

Prevention of External Apical Root Resorption

3

Abstract

The issue of orthodontic-induced external apical root resorption (EARR) has attracted the interest of clinicians and investigators because of the alarming clinical and legal implications associated with its occurrence in a severe form. The January/February 2005 issue of the American Association of Orthodontist's Bulletin reported that medical malpractice is a significant problem in the USA today and that patients are filing claims and lawsuits against medical and dental practitioners, including orthodontists, in record numbers. EARR is a common iatrogenic consequence of orthodontic treatment. Cross-sectional as well as longitudinal studies show that EARR is a small problem for the average orthodontic patient, with radiographic mean resorption of less than 2.5 mm. This magnitude of resorption has no adverse clinical consequences. However, 1–5 % of orthodontic patients experience a severe form of EARR, defined as exceeding 4 mm or one-third of the original root length. Severe root resorption mainly occurs in maxillary incisors. It compromises crown-root ratios and can result in tooth mobility. The main etiologic risk factor for the severe form of EARR is genetic predisposition. Emphasis is thus given on the root-sparing treatment procedures to minimize the risk for development of the severe form of EARR.

3.1 Introduction

Root resorption has been classified by Fuss et al. [1] according to the stimulating factors that induce it. The resorption-stimulating factors include pulpal infection resorption, periodontal infection resorption, ankylotic resorption, impacted tooth or tumor pressure resorption, and orthodontic pressure resorption. *Infection root resorption* can occur either on the internal or the external root surface and is caused by microbial pathogens. *Ankylotic root resorption* is caused by macrophages digesting hyalinized tissue following tooth macro-trauma; injury to the root surface is

R. Justus, *Iatrogenic Effects of Orthodontic Treatment: Decision-Making in Prevention, Diagnosis, and Treatment*, DOI 10.1007/978-3-319-18353-4_3

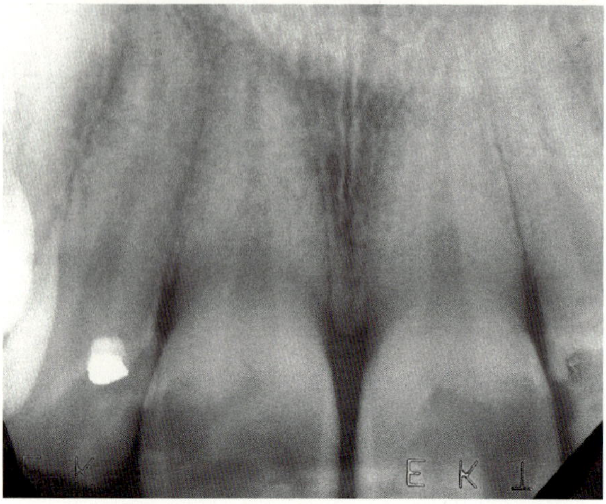

Fig. 3.1 Pretreatment maxillary incisor periapical radiograph of a 36-year-old orthodontic female patient

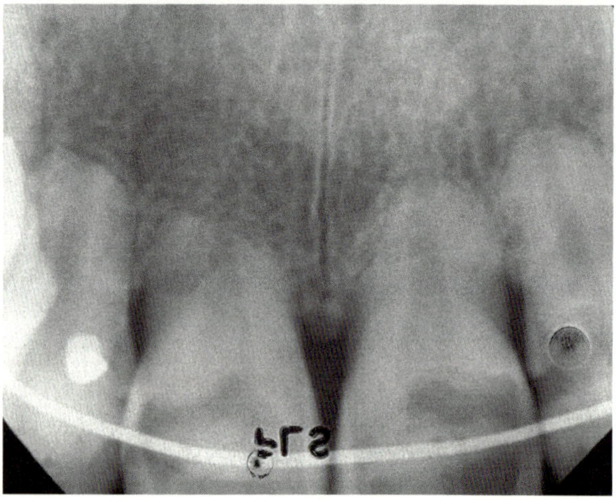

Fig. 3.2 Posttreatment maxillary incisor periapical radiograph of the same patient at age 39. Four bicuspid extraction case. Note severe EARR which required an intracoronal splint due to incisor mobility

usually so large that healing with cementum is not possible; bone is in direct contact with dentin and is laid down without the presence of a periodontal ligament, leading to replacement resorption. *Pressure root resorption* is caused by orthodontic forces or by pressure of impacted teeth or tumors against adjacent roots. Fuss' classification of root resorption allows proper treatment rendering by identifying the stimulating factors.

This chapter will be exclusively dedicated to orthodontic pressure resulting in external apical root resorption (EARR), which is the loss of root structure involving the apical region (Figs. 3.1 and 3.2). The chapter has been divided into seven subchapters which include pathology, epidemiology, risk factors, etiology, prognosis, clinical recommendations to protect patients from developing EARR, and recommendations to minimize or avoid malpractice lawsuits.

3.2 Pathology

The textbook *Contemporary Orthodontics* [2] has an excellent description of the EARR process. For the benefit of the reader, the following is a brief summary.

Frontal resorption of the alveolar lamina dura is a desirable process in orthodontic tooth movement because it is not associated with root resorption, while undermining resorption is an undesirable and pathological process since it is associated with root resorption. Undermining resorption occurs when compression of the periodontal ligament (PDL), produced by a sustained orthodontic force against a tooth, is great enough to totally occlude blood vessels and cut off the blood supply to an area within the PDL. Blood flow impediment results in hyalinization, also known as sterile necrosis. During the initial repair phase of the necrosed areas, clast cells resorb not only the underside of the lamina dura but also the cementum and dentin. Removal of hyalinized tissue leads to removal of cementoid and mature collagen, leaving a raw cemental surface that is readily attacked by dentinoclasts. Once orthodontic movement stops, these root craters usually fill back in with cementum, restoring the original contours of the root. However, if the attack on the root surface produced large defects at the apex, they eventually become separated from the root surface. Once an island of cementum or dentin has been cut totally free from the root surface, it will be resorbed and will not be replaced. Thus, shortening of the root occurs when cavities coalesce at the apex, so that peninsulas of root structure are cut off as islands. Then the repair process smoothes over the new root surface and a net loss of root length occurs. Forces are concentrated at the root apex because orthodontic tooth movement is never entirely translatory, which places the narrow periapical region in harm's way. The coronal third of a root is covered with acellular cementum, whereas the apical third is cellular and the middle third is intermediate. Cellular cementum forms more rapidly and is more active than acellular cementum, but this cellular periapical cementum depends on a patent vasculature. Accordingly, periapical cementum is more friable and easily injured in the face of heavy forces and concomitant vascular stasis. Despite the clinician's best efforts to keep forces light and well distributed to induce only frontal resorption, some areas of undermining resorption are probably produced in every patient [2].

Light forces are precisely what orthodontists have been applying since the late 1970s when brackets welded to bands were replaced by direct bonding. Bonding brackets to enamel obligated orthodontists to diminish the magnitude of applied force by using lighter wires to avoid accidental dislodgement of brackets. Currently, narrower brackets are available in order to increase the interbracket distance, resulting in additional force reduction due to increased wire springiness. Many orthodontists are using .018″ instead of .022″ slot brackets, which also diminishes the magnitude of forces that can be applied. Further, some orthodontists are even using glass ionomer cement to bond brackets to minimize the development of white spot lesions. This type of cement limits even more the magnitude of forces that can be applied, particularly during the first 24 h after bonding, because of the diminished bonding adhesion of this cement when compared to composite resin. If orthodontic force magnitude would be the main cause for severe EARR, the incidence should have diminished dramatically since less force magnitude has been used for the past 40 years (due to the use of direct bonded brackets). Unfortunately, this has not occurred.

3.3 Epidemiology

EARR is a common iatrogenic consequence of orthodontic treatment. In an extensive literature review of the evidence for EARR and orthodontic treatment, Weltman [3] made several critical observations. First, post-orthodontic treatment incidence of EARR is 73 % (detected radiographically). Cross-sectional as well as longitudinal studies show that EARR is a small problem for the average orthodontic patient with a radiographic mean resorption of less than 2.5 mm. This magnitude of resorption has no adverse clinical consequences, but unfortunately, 1–5 % of orthodontic patients experience a severe form of EARR (defined as exceeding 4 mm or one-third of the original root length). Severe root resorption mainly occurs in maxillary incisors followed by mandibular incisors and mandibular first molars. Finally, this magnitude of EARR compromises crown-root ratios and can unfortunately result in tooth mobility. Incisor mobility sometimes requires splinting (Fig. 3.2).

More recent studies [4–9] investigating EARR incidence and comparing the severity with lighter forces and studies [10–12] investigating heavier forces, used before the introduction of direct bonding, show similar results. The conclusion is that development of EARR may not necessarily be due to the degree of applied orthodontic force per se but also to a patient's individual genetic predisposition or susceptibility.

3.4 Risk Factors

Many factors have been proposed as risk factors for the appearance of the severe form of EARR. These can be divided into orthodontic treatment-related risk factors and patient-related risk factors [13]. Examples of treatment-related risk factors are treatment duration [14–25], magnitude of applied force [19, 26–31], direction of tooth movement [11, 24, 25, 27, 32–35], amount of apical displacement [16, 21], method of force application (continuous vs. intermittent) [12, 28, 36–41], type of appliance [42–44], and treatment technique [24, 32, 44–53].

Examples of risk factors related to the patient include previous history of EARR [42, 54–56]; tooth-root morphology, length, and roots with developmental abnormalities [4, 7, 9, 11, 21–23, 57–63]; genetic influences [7, 54, 64–68]; systemic factors [69–72] including drugs (nabumetone) [73]; hormone deficiency, hypothyroidism, and hypopituitarism [74–77]; asthma [41, 58]; root proximity to cortical bone [11, 15, 78]; alveolar bone density [15, 79–81]; chronic alcoholism [82]; previous trauma [9, 12, 41, 47, 54–56, 83–85]; endodontic treatment [4, 10, 35, 41, 55,

56, 86]; severity and type of malocclusion [4, 7–9, 11, 16, 17, 20, 31, 54, 87]; and patient age [12, 14, 17, 21, 22, 36, 88–92], patient gender [7, 17, 21, 31, 56, 57, 65, 78, 93], and patient habits [94].

Most researchers agree that all of the identified risk factors only explain a small percentage of the variation in EARR. In 1998, Vlaskalic [95] stated: "The long list of suspected causative factors for EARR highlights the state of ignorance that exists with respect to EARR and orthodontic treatment." Fortunately, more light has been shed since then on the etiology of EARR. Årtun et al. [96], in 2005, reported the results of a multicenter clinical study on EARR in which maxillary incisor periapical radiographs were obtained in 302 consecutively treated orthodontic patients who had fixed appliances. The radiographs were taken at three time periods: pretreatment and 6 and 12 months after appliance placement. The result was that orthodontic patients with detectable EARR during the first 6 months of active treatment are more likely to experience resorption in the following 6-month period than those without such exhibited early EARR. These authors concluded that the low explained variance of identified risk factors, combined with the strong association between the amount of EARR during the first and second 6-month treatment period, suggested a genetic predisposition as the major etiologic factor.

It can be concluded from this study that it is critical for clinicians to obtain periapical radiographs of maxillary incisors 6 months after fixed appliance placement *of every patient* to identify patients at risk of further EARR.

3.5 Etiology

EARR is apparently related to a genetic predisposition. Harris et al. [65], in a study using the sib-pair model, reported that the strongest single association with EARR seems to be a person's genotype since familial studies showed that a person's genotype accounts for about two-thirds of the variation in the extent of EARR. These authors concluded that an individual's genetic background is the single strongest predictor of EARR, as shown by familial analysis. The first report, in which a genetic marker was described identifying people who are susceptible to EARR before beginning orthodontic treatment, was published by Al-Qawasmi et al. [64]. This paper, titled "Genetic predisposition to EARR," investigated whether there is linkage and association between polymorphisms of the interleukin IL-1 genes and EARR. The sample consisted of 35 white American families. Each family included two or more siblings treated with orthodontics. Genomic DNA was obtained for isolation and analysis from buccal swab cells of the siblings and their parents. Highly significant evidence of linkage disequilibrium of IL-1B polymorphism with EARR in the maxillary central incisors was obtained. Persons carrying two alleles # 1 (one from the father, the other from the mother) of the IL-1B have, on average, 1.3 mm more EARR than those with either the alleles 1 and 2 or the alleles 2 and 2. Persons homozygous for the IL-1B allele # 1 have a 5.6-fold increased risk of EARR greater than 2 mm as compared with those who are not homozygous for the IL-1B allele 1. When the

EARR value of 2 mm was used to divide subjects into affected and unaffected, 72 % of EARR occurred in those carrying both alleles # 1, followed by 39 % of EARR in those carrying the two different alleles, 1 and 2, and 0 % incidence in individuals carrying the two protective alleles # 2. Thus, data indicate that allele 1 and the IL-1B gene, known to decrease the production of IL-1 cytokine in vivo, significantly increase the risk of EARR. The authors propose a model for the pathway through which IL-1B genotype modulates the extent of EARR experienced during orthodontic tooth movement. Their hypothesis is that low IL-1B production in the case of allele 1 results in less catabolic bone modeling in the cortical bone interface of PDL because of decreased number of osteoclasts associated with lower levels of this cytokine. Inhibition of bone resorption in the direction of tooth movement results in maintaining prolonged dynamic loading of tooth root adjacent to compressed PDL, resulting in more EARR because of fatigue failure of the root. In the case of high IL-1B production associated with allele 2, compressed PDL space is restored by resorption of bone interface of PDL, resulting in only mild EARR that is controlled by the cementum-healing mechanism. In spite of the authors' encouraging findings that EARR does indeed have a genetic basis, they concluded that the genetic predictors of EARR are not yet reliable because IL-1B polymorphism accounts for only 15 % of the total variation of maxillary incisor EARR. These authors report that many genes besides IL-1B are probably involved, that a search for the remaining genetic factors that influence EARR is ongoing with the ultimate goal of providing orthodontic treatment that circumvents EARR, and that in the future DNA analysis might provide a more accurate risk assessment for EARR.

3.6 Prognosis

This subtopic is subdivided into pretreatment, active treatment, and posttreatment prognosis.

3.6.1 Pretreatment Prognosis

Harris et al. [65] (previously mentioned) suggested that an individual's genetic background could assist in doing an EARR pretreatment risk assessment. These authors recommended that post-orthodontic radiographs of siblings and/or parents be evaluated to predict risk for EARR. In other words, a prior sibling's orthodontic outcome could be a useful gauge of another sibling's risk of EARR. Unfortunately, sibling and parent's posttreatment radiographs are not frequently available.

3.6.2 Active Treatment Prognosis

When EARR is detected during orthodontic treatment, it will progress for as long as the treatment continues, as demonstrated by (Årtun et al. [96]). Patients should be made aware of the problem. If the decision is to continue orthodontic treatment, further radiographic monitoring of the patient is recommended. Also, even lighter forces should be applied and alternate upper and lower arch wire activations, for example, activating once every 2–3 months each individual arch instead of monthly. Rest periods are thus built into treatment. The teeth are orthodontically moved, followed by a period during which forces are minimized with passive arch wires for 2–3 months to allow root repair. Movement could then be resumed. Therefore, the rate of tooth movement is slowed, and the reparative process of the cementum can keep abreast of the erosive processes of over-compression of the PDL, as the root is forced against the alveolus. A force-free rest period allows the cementum to recover the exposed dentin, thus improving root length at the end of treatment. A pause also permits repair of the necrotic hyalinization zone, including central tissue zones in the PDL that appear to be protective of the root. Levander et al. [97], in 1994, reported a clinical study evaluating the effect of a treatment pause on teeth in which EARR was discovered after an initial treatment period of 6 months with fixed appliances. They found that the amount of EARR was significantly less in patients treated with a pause of 2–3 months than it was in patients treated without interruption.

3.6.3 Posttreatment Prognosis

Once the patient is in the retention phase, EARR ceases [10] and root healing processes occur, such as remodeling of irregular apical areas, apical rounding, smoothing of edges, and return to a normal PDL width. Statistical modeling has shown that 3 mm of apical root loss equates to 20 % loss of attachment area and that 1 mm of crestal bone loss also creates 20 % loss of attachment [98]. Thus, conservation of crestal bone level is paramount when EARR occurs. To improve post-orthodontic treatment prognosis, occlusal equilibration to eliminate interferences is recommended. If tooth mobility is present, an intracoronal stabilizer should be bonded (similar to a canine to canine fixed retainer). In addition, maintenance of excellent oral hygiene and frequent dental appointments for professional prophylaxis are recommended.

3.7 Clinical Recommendations to Protect Patients from Developing EARR

Since orthodontists cannot yet identify which pre-orthodontic patients are susceptible to severe EARR, a signed informed consent is important both for adequate patient education and for proper risk management. Dental histories reporting macro-trauma should alert the clinician because there is an increased risk of EARR associated with macro-trauma [83]. The clinician should also be aware that teeth with short roots have an increased risk of loss in patients who also have crestal alveolar bone height loss [98], particularly if the roots have been shortened even more by EARR. In susceptible patients, the probability of EARR development in its severe form is increased by the following: moving teeth considerable distances [16, 21], using heavy continuous orthodontic forces [19, 26–31], moving teeth that have had previous macro-trauma [83], moving teeth against cortical plates [11, 15, 78] (as is frequently done in patients with severe skeletal discrepancies treated with orthodontics exclusively instead of a combination of orthodontics and orthognathic surgery), and an increased treatment time [14–25]. Specifically, patients who need orthognathic surgery to achieve a successful result, but are treated nonsurgically, usually take longer to treat. Long and narrow roots are also at increased risk for EARR since in tipping movements, the longer the root, the more pressure at the root apex due to longer moment arms. EARR can be minimized in orthodontic patients by moving teeth with light forces, through trabecular bone, with periodic radiographic monitoring and, most importantly, by moving them the least distance possible. This may be accomplished by using the following root-sparing orthodontic treatment regimes:

1. Growth modification to correct severe skeletal Class II malocclusions
2. Early interception of maxillary canines that have mesial eruption paths
3. Serial extraction to modify eruption paths (guidance of eruption)
4. Correction of anterior open bite with a palatal tongue spur appliance
5. Orthognathic surgery to avoid moving teeth large distances and against cortical plates

The ultimate goal of these five recommended treatment strategies is to provide orthodontic treatment that circumvents EARR. The following are clinical examples of some of these regimes.

3.7.1 Growth Modification to Correct Severe Skeletal Class II Malocclusions

There is considerable controversy among orthodontists about the timing of orthodontic treatment. Those who promote early treatment in the mixed dentition claim to have better results, even though a second phase of orthodontic treatment may be required. Some orthodontists however prefer to initiate treatment in the late mixed dentition with the belief that they can achieve equally good clinical results in a single phase. This section presents a case report of a Class II, Division 1 patient that significantly benefited from early mixed dentition treatment. Emphasis on early treatment helps to achieve lip competence, prevent incisor fractures, diminish the need for extraction of permanent teeth, and minimize the possibility of EARR. The recommended appliances are shown, as well as the long-term clinical results and stability.

Advantages of early treatment should include the following:

- Early/timely Class II treatment helps to minimize incisor trauma and external apical root resorption.
- Prevention of incisor tooth trauma helps avoid its long-term consequences.
- Combination headgear is superior to functional appliances.

- Utilization of all the growth accelerations that occur in growing patients rather than just the adolescent growth acceleration is advantageous.
- Maxillary sutural growth can be easily modified while mandibular growth cannot.
- Differential growth is the key to long-term stability.
- Children's compliance is better than adolescent's as documented by timing devices [99].

Children with severe skeletal Class II, Division 1 malocclusions, with large overjets, may be treated using their growth potential by inhibiting maxillary growth while mandibular downward and forward growth takes place. Taking advantage of growth to correct an overjet minimizes the need for extensive tooth movement (avoids dental compensations). Therefore, risk of the development of EARR is diminished. In addition, trauma to the incisors may be prevented when lip incompetence due to Class II malocclusion is treated in the early mixed dentition [100–104].

Class II skeletal correction is likely best achieved through the use of a combination occipito-cervical headgear. Functional appliances accomplish Class II correction mostly through tooth movement (proclination of mandibular incisors and retroclination of maxillary incisors) [105, 106], thereby increasing the risk of EARR in genetically susceptible patients. Also, the probability of bicuspid extractions is increased when Class II malocclusion correction is achieved with functional appliances because these appliances tend to procline lower incisors [106, 107]. This proclination, as reviewed in Chap. 2 of this book, compromises *long-term stability*, *periodontal health*, and facial *esthetics*.

In the practice of orthodontics, we as specialists have to decide, among many things, whether a patient requires extraction or non-extraction therapy taking into account the magnitude of dental crowding in the setting of the patient's initial facial profile. When functional appliances are used to correct Class II malocclusions, the probability of requiring extraction of bicuspids is higher because both fixed and removable functional appliances tend to procline lower incisors. The evidence that lower incisors procline with the use of functional appliances is given by the randomized clinical trials of early Class II treatment published by O'Brien et al. [106] and by Tulloch et al. [107]. The latter study found that 31 % of a group of patients treated in the mixed dentition with a functional appliance (modified bionator) eventually required bicuspid extractions compared with a group of patients who used a combination headgear in which the extraction rate was only 16 %. Patient E serves as an example of how a skeletal Class II malocclusion was corrected in a growing child with the use of a headgear. The patient did not require extraction therapy in the second phase of treatment because proclination of lower incisors did not occur as would have arisen with the use of a functional appliance.

Patient E, treated by the author, illustrates the advantages of using a combination (occipital and cervical traction) headgear to correct a *skeletal* Class II, Division 1 malocclusion. Correction of a large incisor overjet by growth modification with a headgear avoided having to move incisors thereby protecting them from experiencing EARR. Headgear use also helped avoid the need for extractions in the second phase of treatment because lower incisors were not proclined, a factor also minimizing risk of EARR.

Patient E was a 6.0-year-old healthy girl (Figs. 3.3, 3.4, and 3.5) with a skeletal Class II, Division 1 subdivision malocclusion (Fig. 3.6) with lip incompetence. She exhibited a protrusive maxillary lip, a lower lip trapped behind her maxillary incisors, and a retrusive mandible. Her maxilla was prognathic, and her mandible was retrognathic with an ANB angle of 10° (SNA 85°, SNB 75°). Her vertical relationships were within normal limits, with a mandibular plane to SN angle of 35° (Fig. 3.7). Her lower incisors were slightly protrusive both relative to her mandibular plane (100°) and to her NB line (+5 mm). Her maxillary incisors were somewhat retrusive being 2 mm in front of the NA line but normal relative to the SN line, being at an angle of 102°. She had an 11.5-mm anterior overjet (Figs. 3.8, 3.9, 3.10, and 3.11) and a normal overbite. Her lower incisors were crowded (Fig. 3.12) with the lower dental midline deviated 2 mm to the right of her maxillary dental midline (Fig. 3.9). The molar relationships were end-to-end Class II on the right side (Fig. 3.8) and Class I on the left side (Fig. 3.10).

A combination headgear was recommended to correct the overjet by maxillary forward growth inhibition and naturally occurring mandibular forward growth. Lip incompetence would self-correct with the abovementioned maxillary growth modification. The mixed dentition analysis revealed that all permanent teeth would be able to erupt with sufficient space if leeway space was held. In addition, serial extraction of the primary teeth would be required, starting with extraction of her two primary mandibular canines to allow self-alignment (driftodontics) of her crowded lower incisors. As soon as these incisors self-aligned (by tongue pressure alone), a mandibular lingual holding arch would be cemented on her lower first permanent molars. The patient and her parents were also informed that full fixed appliances might later be required following the eruption of all of her permanent teeth to do the final detailing of the occlusion and to achieve proper dental alignment. Both the patient and her parents accepted the treatment plan.

Treatment objectives were to change the facial profile from maxillary prognathic and mandibular retrognathic to orthognathic, to reduce the anterior overjet, to achieve lip competence, and to align the lower incisors. Maxillo-mandibular growth was expected in this patient since she was a 6-year-old female with her menarche still years away. A combination headgear was recommended to inhibit maxillary horizontal growth while mandibular growth proceeded, hopefully, in a forward and downward direction.

The combination headgear (Fig. 3.13) delivers two simultaneous and equal forces to the maxillary first permanent molars, a cervical distal force and an occipital distal force. The resultant vector of these two simultaneous forces is a horizontal distal force (Fig. 3.14). The objective of applying these two forces is to provide a distalizing force through the molars that will not extrude nor intrude them. These forces, if they are of orthopedic magnitude (400 g per side), modify the growth direction of the maxillofacial sutures [108–114]. The line of action of the force should ideally pass horizontally through the center of resistance of the molars in order to avoid tipping them. This can be achieved by raising the outer bow so that the line of action of the two forces passes through the center of resistance of the molars which is considered to be located at the

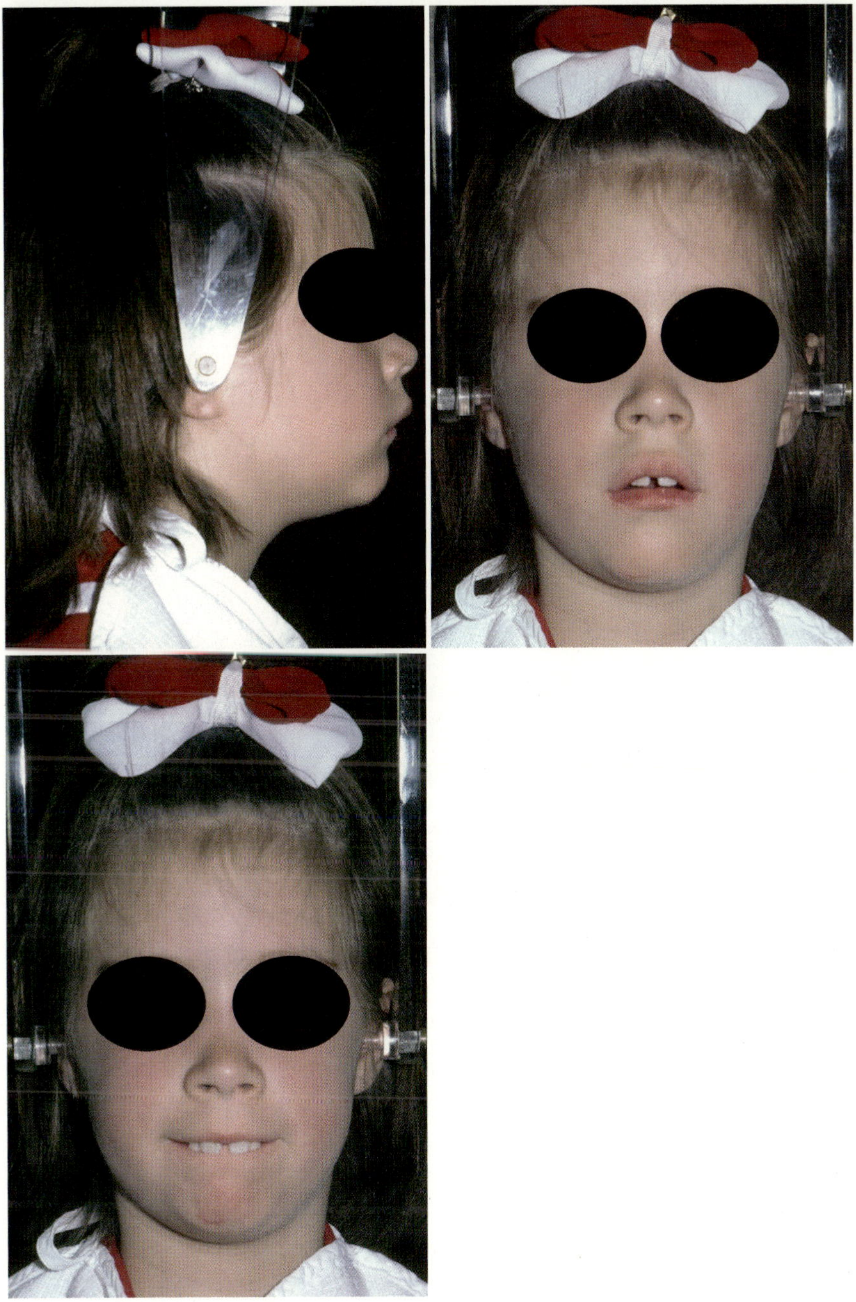

Figs. 3.3, 3.4, and 3.5 Pretreatment facial photographs of a 6-year-old female patient. Note Class II profile with a protrusive upper lip and a retrusive lower lip associated with a large ANB angle (10°). Also note incompetent lips

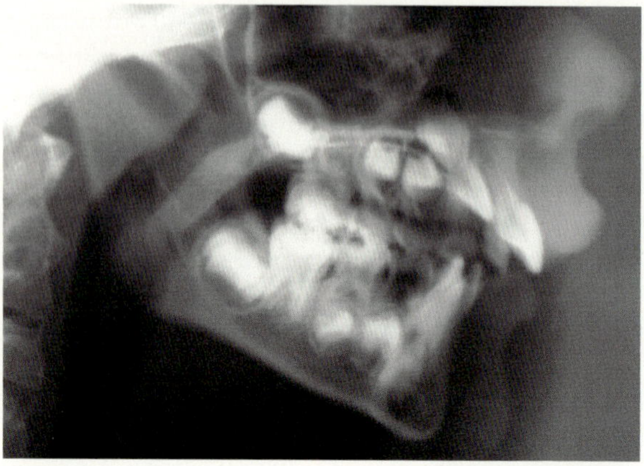

Fig. 3.6 Pretreatment close-up of cephalogram. Note large incisor overjet (11.5 mm) due to a retrognathic mandible (SNB 75°) and a prognathic maxilla (SNA 85°), with the lower lip trapped behind the maxillary incisors

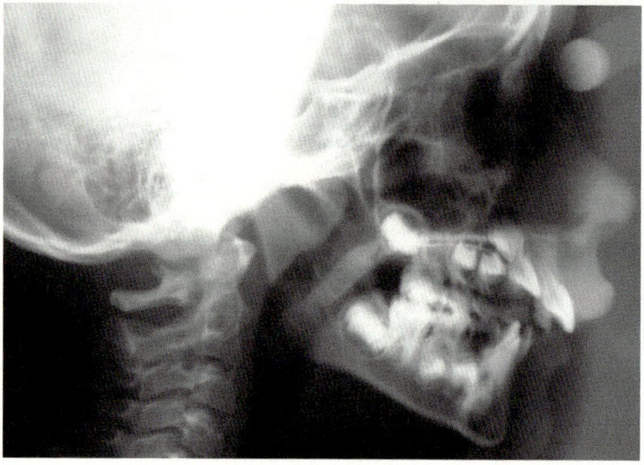

Fig. 3.7 Pretreatment cephalogram. Mandibular plane angle to SN is 35°, giving normal vertical proportions

level of their trifurcation. The maxillary first permanent molars are used as anchors to transmit the orthopedic forces to the maxillary sutures to restrict their horizontal growth rather than to distalize the molars themselves. Even though the molars move distally while the headgear is worn (nighttime), they migrate to their original positions when the headgear is not being worn (usually daytime); the net effect is skeletal modification exclusively, not dental movement. The outer bow should be short, with its distal end coinciding with the anteroposterior position of the anchor molars. The inner bow should be expanded by 2 mm symmetrically so that when it is placed in one molar tube, it rests just outside the other tube. This should be done during the monthly appointments because the relative forward growth of the mandible will produce a posterior crossbite tendency, unless the upper arch width is expanded.

The patient was given a combination headgear (Fig. 3.13) at age 6.0 with instructions to wear it unfailingly every night and, when possible, afternoons also. Her mixed dentition analysis predicted that all her permanent teeth mesial to the first molars would be able to erupt with sufficient space, without the need to increase arch length. Her mandibular primary canines were extracted to allow the permanent

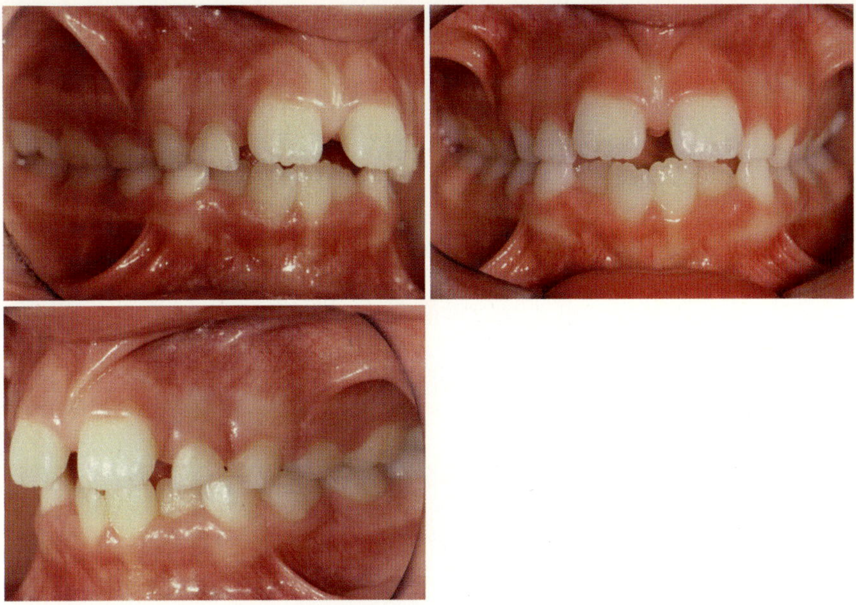

Figs. 3.8, 3.9, and 3.10 Pretreatment intraoral views with teeth in occlusion. Note end-to-end Class II malocclusion on the right side and Class I on the left side, with mandibular dental midline deviated toward the right side. Also note crowding of lower incisors and a maxillary central incisor diastema

Fig. 3.11 Pretreatment dental casts in occlusion reveal the 11.5-mm incisor overjet

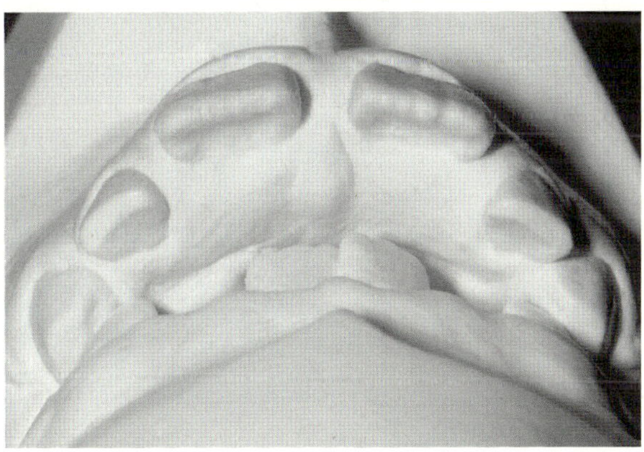

lateral incisors to be aligned by tongue pressure. Three months after the extractions, the lateral incisors were sufficiently aligned (Fig. 3.15) to allow the placement of a fixed lingual holding arch (Fig. 3.16). One year later, the lower first primary molars were extracted (Fig. 3.17) to allow the permanent canines to erupt with sufficient space (Fig. 3.18). Eighteen months later, the lower second primary molars were extracted (Fig. 3.19) to allow the first and second bicuspids to erupt taking

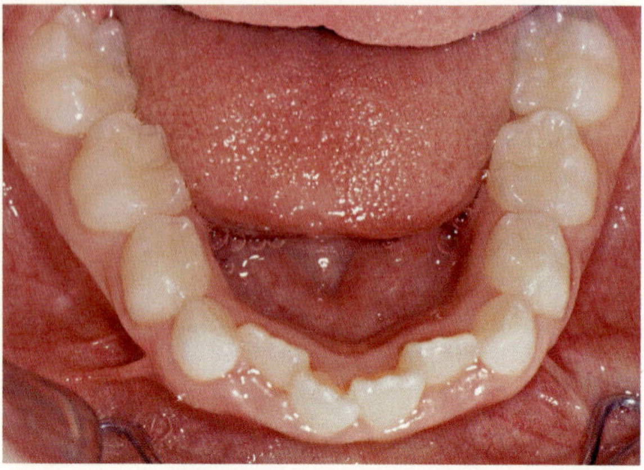

Fig. 3.12 Pretreatment intraoral mandibular occlusal view. Note a 4-mm arch length deficiency without taking into account the leeway space

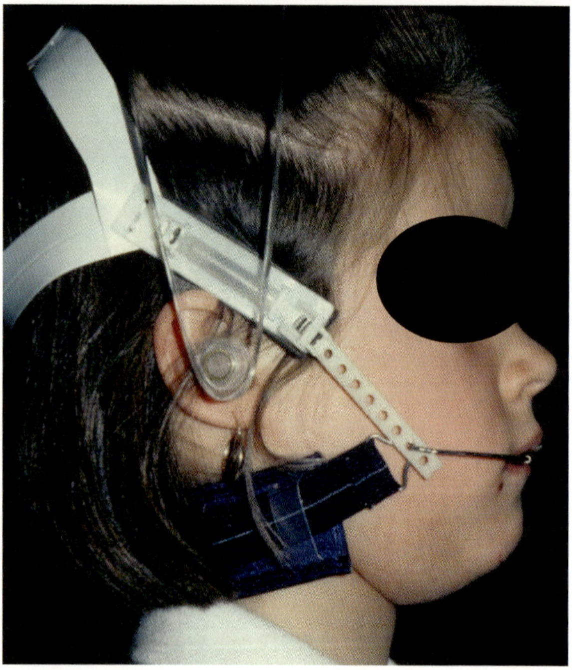

Fig. 3.13 Combination headgear used to restrain maxillary sutural growth in a forward direction while natural mandibular growth proceeds downward and forward

advantage of the leeway space. Once all her permanent lower teeth erupted, brackets were bonded to all her lower permanent teeth (Fig. 3.20) to correct minor rotations (Fig. 3.21). Four months later, she was debonded (Fig. 3.22) and the headgear was discontinued. A lower removable retainer (Fig. 3.23) and a maxillary removable wraparound retainer were given to the patient along with instructions to wear them every night for as long as she wished to keep her teeth well aligned. Final records were taken, and the patient was asked to return annually for retainer checkups and to observe whether the third molars would erupt in a correct position.

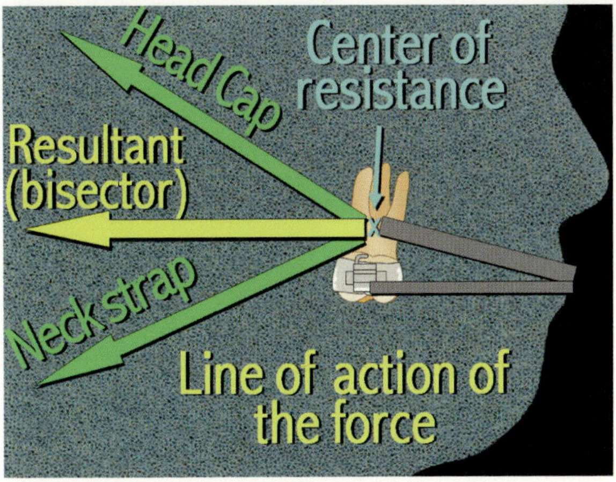

Fig. 3.14 Diagram illustrating the forces and vectors associated with the combination headgear. The objective of the two applied forces (cervical and occipital) on the maxillary first molars is to use them as anchors to transmit these forces to the maxillofacial sutures, inhibiting maxillary forward growth (growth modification)

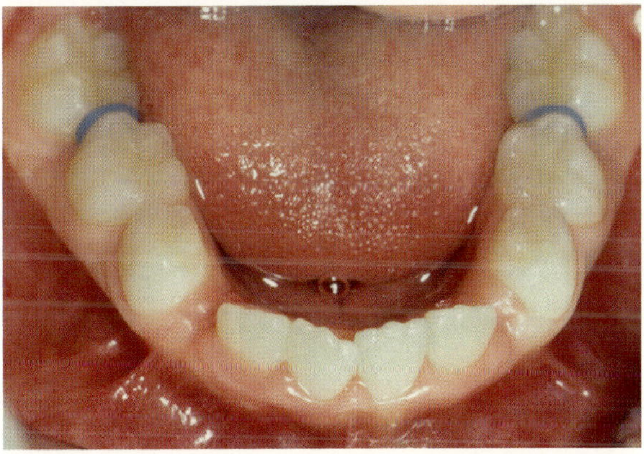

Fig. 3.15 Three months post-extraction of primary lower canines, progress view at age 6.3. Note that the lateral incisors are in better alignment having been moved forward by tongue pressure. Blue Alastik separators were placed mesial to the lower first permanent molars to create band space for a cemented lingual holding arch

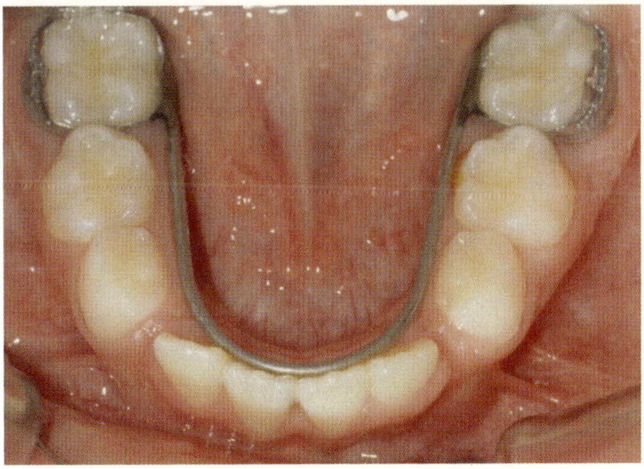

Fig. 3.16 Lower holding arch cemented

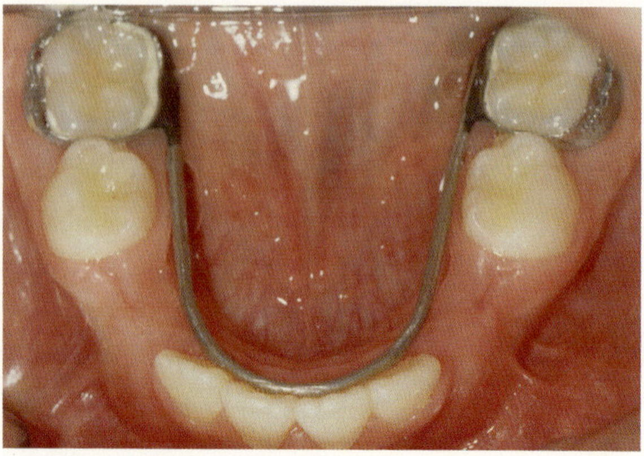

Fig. 3.17 Extraction of lower first primary molars to give space for the erupting canines. Progress view

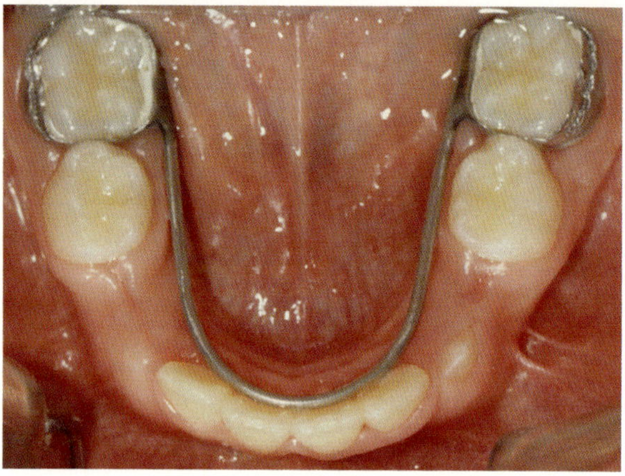

Fig. 3.18 Progress view of erupting canines

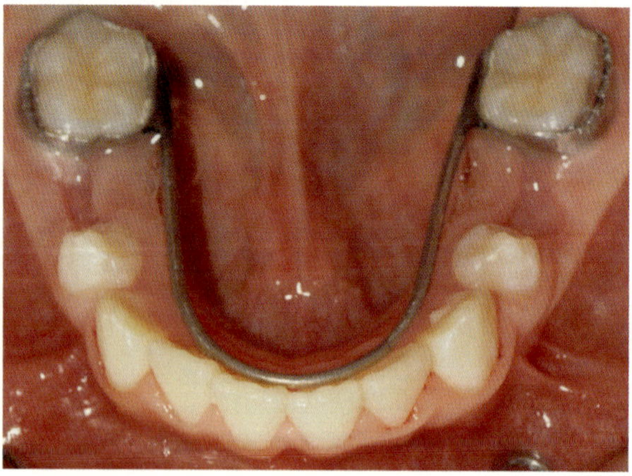

Fig. 3.19 Extraction of second primary molars to give space for the eruption of the first and second premolars using the leeway space

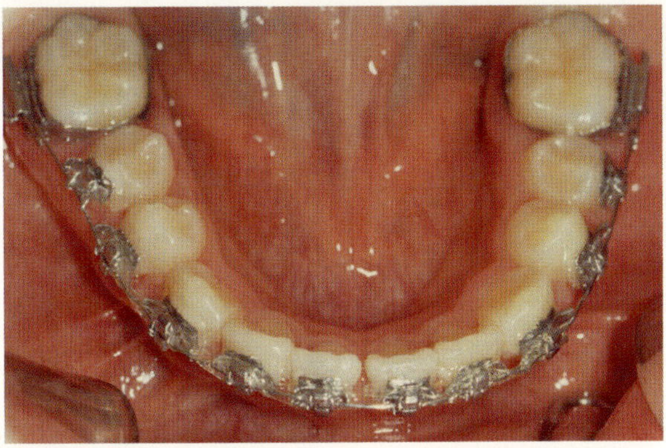

Fig. 3.20 Brackets bonded to all lower teeth for final alignment detailing

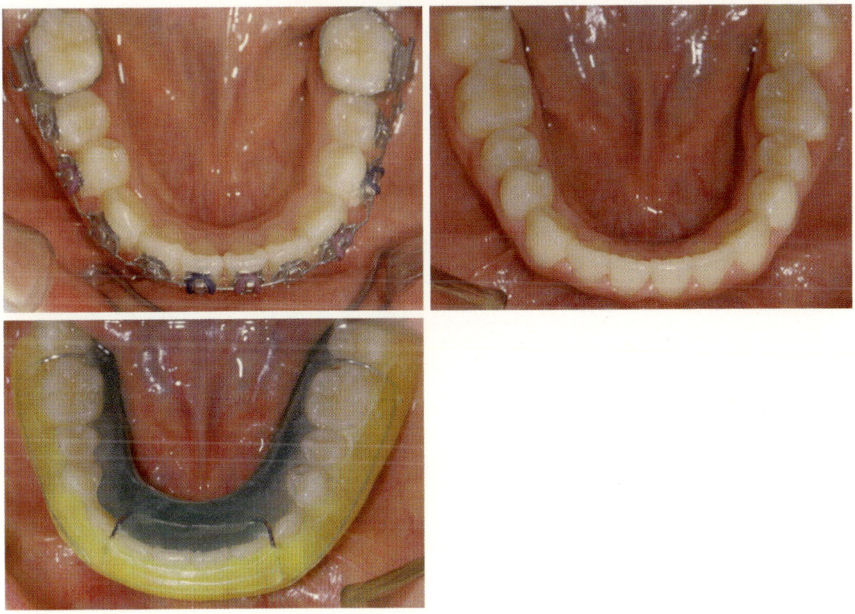

Figs. 3.21, 3.22, and 3.23 Detailing finished. Brackets were debonded and a removable retainer was given to the patient. Note good dental alignment at age 11.5

The optimal maxillary retainer is the wraparound type. The reason for using this type of retainer is that the labial/buccal wire does not interfere with the occlusion. The lower retainer design can be seen in Fig. 3.23. It is a retainer that covers both the labial and the lingual of all the teeth in the arch. This retainer impedes labiolingual and rotational tooth movements from occurring and also impedes extraction spaces from reopening, in cases in which extractions were required [115].

Progress facial profile photographs taken during treatment document the changes as they arose during treatment (Figs. 3.24, 3.25, 3.26, and 3.27). Posttreatment facial frontal views demonstrate lip competence and a pleasing smile (Figs. 3.28

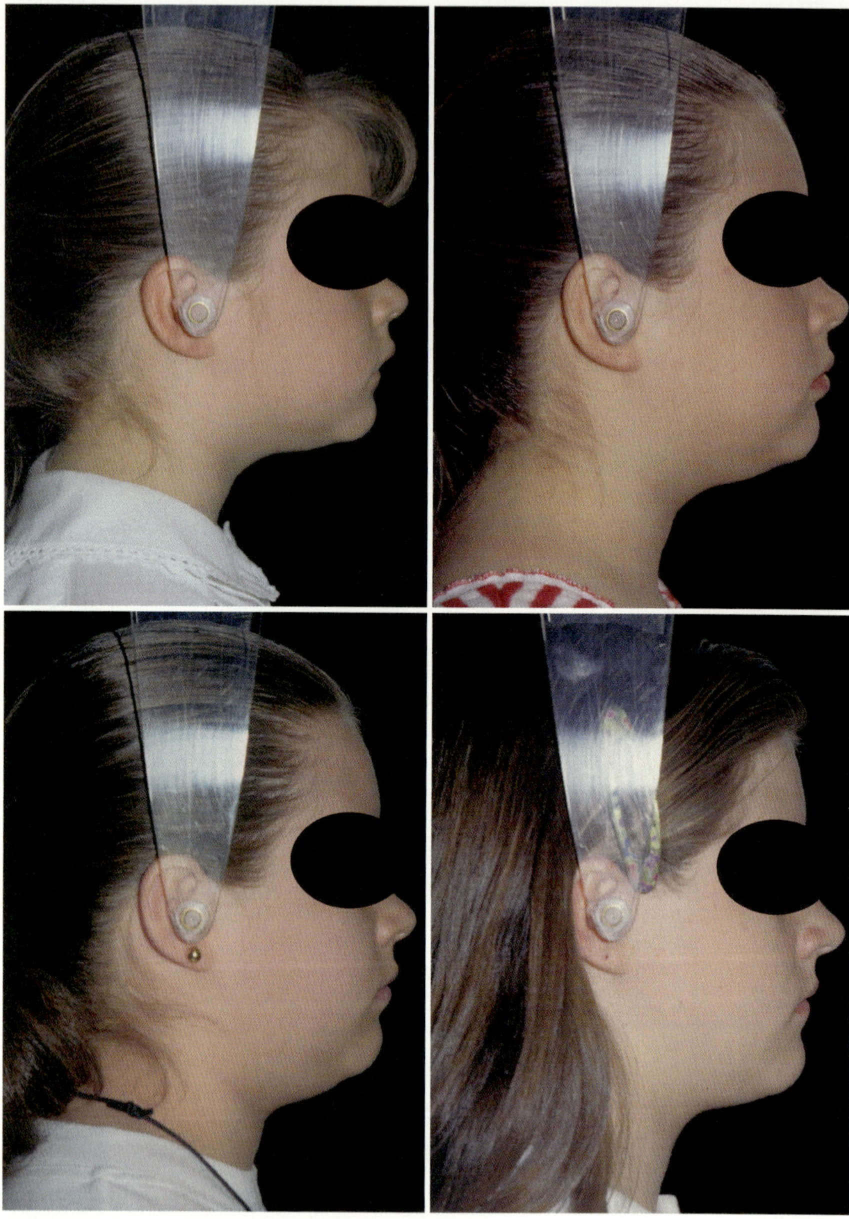

Figs. 3.24, 3.25, 3.26, and 3.27 Progress facial profile views (ages 8.0, 9.0, 10.0, and 11.5) showing the gradual improvement from a typical Class II to a Class I face. These dramatic changes occurred due to the patient's excellent cooperation with headgear use and the good mandibular growth pattern the patient exhibited. Note the pleasing final profile result. This was due to an increased chin projection and a decreased maxillary lip protrusion, which resulted in lip competence

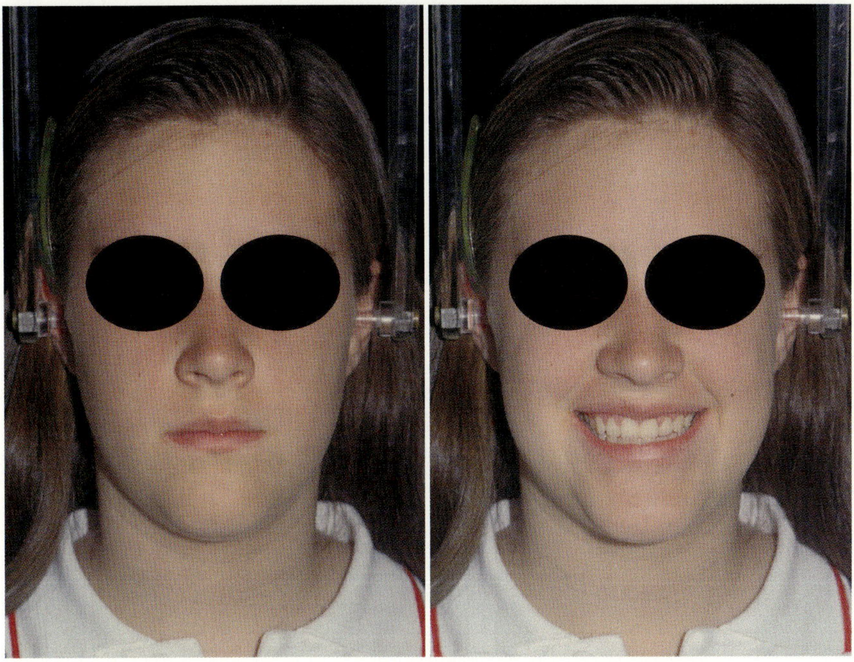

Figs. 3.28 and 3.29 Posttreatment facial frontal views. Note good lip competence and a pleasing smile with the lower lip in consonance with the maxillary incisal borders and the full length of the maxillary teeth being exhibited

and 3.29). Progress intraoral lateral photographs of the right side with teeth in occlusion also document the same features intraorally (Figs. 3.30, 3.31, 3.32, 3.33, and 3.34). It can be observed in Fig. 3.31 that during treatment with the headgear, maxillary brackets were bonded to her four maxillary incisors to close a central incisor diastema. These brackets were removed 4 months later once the diastema was closed.

The patient and her parents were very pleased with the treatment results. Dramatic facial improvements are seen by comparing the pre- and posttreatment photographs (Figs. 3.3, 3.4, and 3.5 with Figs. 3.27, 3.28, and 3.29), the pre- and posttreatment intraoral photographs (Figs. 3.8, 3.9, and 3.10 with Figs. 3.34, 3.35, and 3.36), and the pre- and posttreatment headfilms (Figs. 3.7 and 3.37). The cranial base superimposition of headfilm tracings ages 6.0 and 11.5 (Fig. 3.38) demonstrates that excellent mandibular growth occurred in both direction and magnitude. The forward and downward natural mandibular growth helped to project her originally deficient mandible while the maxilla was restrained in its forward growth. The tracing also demonstrates excellent headgear cooperation because the maxilla was inhibited from growing forward allowing correction of the anterior overjet through mandibular forward growth. The lip incompetence was corrected by restricting maxillary forward growth and by natural mandibular forward growth.

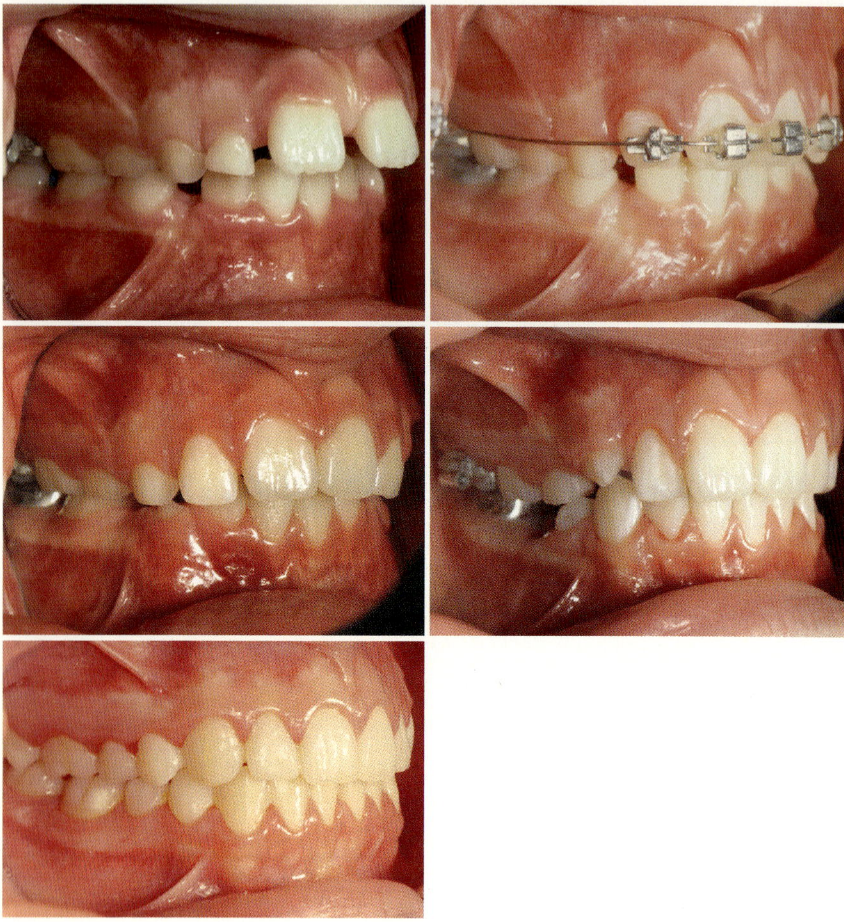

Figs. 3.30, 3.31, 3.32, 3.33, and 3.34 Progress intraoral right side views of teeth in occlusion show the gradual improvement from Class II to Class I (ages 7.0, 8.0, 9.0, and 11.5). These changes occurred due to the patient's excellent cooperation with headgear use and the good growth pattern the patient exhibited. Note the excellent occlusion achieved. This was due to natural mandibular growth while maxilla was being restrained in its forward growth, as shown in Fig. 3.38

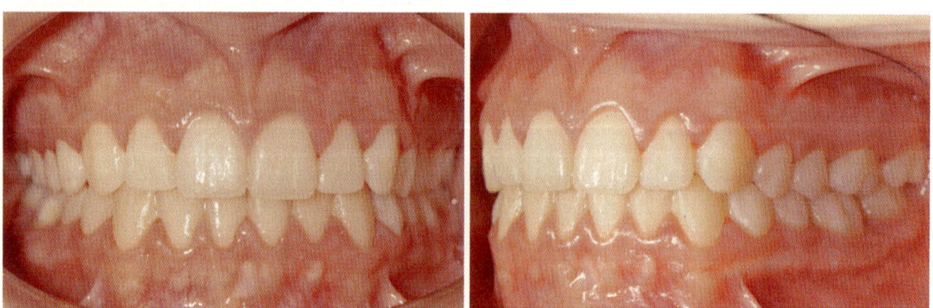

Figs. 3.35 and 3.36 Posttreatment intraoral front and lateral views. Note good occlusion and midline coincidence

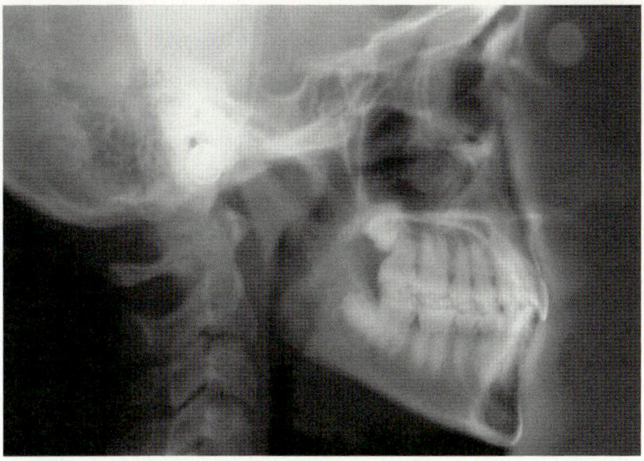

Fig. 3.37 Posttreatment cephalogram. ANB angle is now 3° instead of the original 10°. Note corrected overjet with lower incisors in good position (4 mm in front of the NB line and 88° relative to the mandibular plane). Also note good position of maxillary incisors (3 mm forward of the NA line and 102° relative to the SN line). No dental compensations were required since maxilla and mandible have a normal relationship and lip competence was achieved

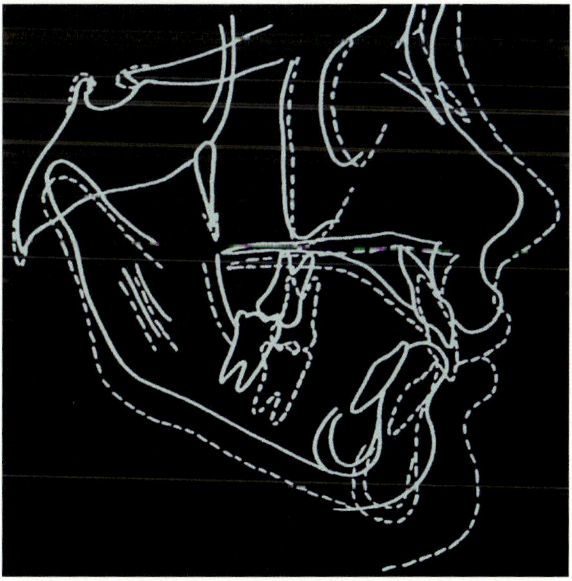

Fig. 3.38 Cranial base superimposition of cephalogram tracings, ages 6.0 and 11.5. Note forward and downward natural mandibular growth while maxillary forward growth was restrained due to good headgear cooperation. Note lip incompetence at age 6.0 and competence at age 11.5

Both maxillary and mandibular cephalometric superimpositions (Figs. 3.39 and 3.40, respectively), ages 6.0 and 11.5, demonstrate no anteroposterior movement of incisors, just continued eruption. No increase in arch length occurred. These excellent incisor positions allowed the lips to have a normal posture and a good facial esthetic outcome.

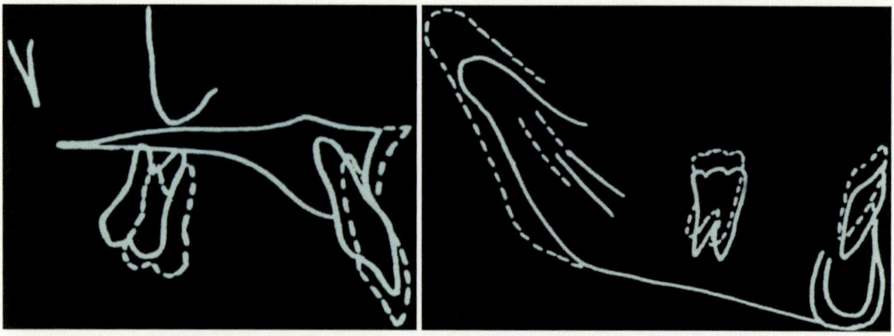

Figs. 3.39 and 3.40 Maxillary and mandibular cephalometric superimpositions of tracings, ages 6.0 and 11.5. Note that maxillary incisors were not retroclined nor lower incisors proclined. The incisors only erupted to compensate the normal skeletal vertical development

Koroluk et al. [101] found that 29.1 % individuals from a sample of orthodontically untreated Class II children with overjets equal or greater than 7 mm had already suffered dental trauma by the age of 9. No incisor trauma occurred in patient E which can be attributed to the *early* correction of the overjet resulting in lip competence. Also, no maxillary incisor EARR occurred in this patient (Figs. 3.41 and 3.42), likely because these teeth themselves were not moved to reduce the overjet. The Class II correction was achieved exclusively through natural mandibular growth while restricting maxillary forward growth.

Patient E returned for a retention visit 6 years posttreatment at the age of 17.6. She exhibited excellent stability of the Class II correction. Full orthodontic records were obtained (Figs. 3.43, 3.44, 3.45, 3.46, 3.47, 3.48, and 3.49). Continued observation of the third molar eruption was recommended. Posttreatment cranial base superimposition of headfilm tracings of ages 11.5 and 17.6 (Fig. 3.50) shows that both the maxilla and the mandible grew downward and forward with the mandible exhibiting a greater magnitude of growth. In addition, more chin soft tissue appeared at the chin in the 6-year posttreatment facial profile photograph (Fig. 3.43). While excellent results were achieved in this case, not all patients grow in such a favorable direction and magnitude, and one must also be aware that the results depend on good patient compliance.

Fidler et al. [116] carried out a study to evaluate the long-term stability of Class II, Division 1 correction. The sample consisted of 78 successfully treated Class II adolescent patients that were evaluated 14 years postretention. The researchers found that the cases that demonstrated long-term stability were those in which the correction was achieved through *differential growth*. They concluded that successful correction of Angle Class II, Division 1 cases through differential growth appears to be very stable. The researchers speculated that growing patients with normal vertical relationships are conducive to good treatment results and long-term stability. Thus, the excellent stability of the Class II correction exhibited by patient E can be attributed to the initial treatment strategy achieved through *differential growth (orthopedics)*, not through dental movements (orthodontics).

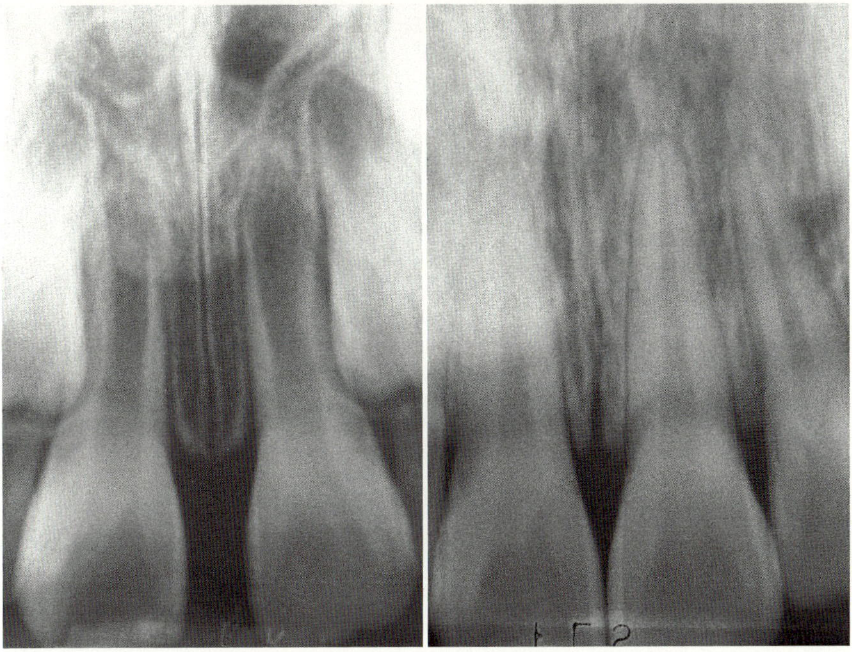

Figs. 3.41 and 3.42 Periapical radiographs taken at ages 6.0 and 11.5. Note continued root development with no trace of EARR, most probably because these teeth were not moved to correct the skeletal Class II or to achieve lip competency

3.7.2 Early Interception of Maxillary Canines with Mesial Eruption Paths

Another orthodontic root-sparing treatment regime involves the early interception of maxillary canines with mesial eruption paths. By extracting the maxillary primary canines [117], and the maxillary first primary molars [118], the eruption path of the permanent canines can frequently be improved and thereby prevent EARR, particularly of the permanent lateral incisors. A preferred strategy is to employ a maxillary removable space holding acrylic plate to prevent the incisors from spacing and also to maintain the extraction spaces open while the canines erupt. Monitoring the eruption path of the canines is critical. The author recommends obtaining panoramic radiographs every 6 months to determine whether potentially impacted canines are responding by modification of their eruption paths. The following case report of patient F illustrates this root-sparing treatment regime.

Patient F was a 9.11-year-old healthy boy with a straight profile (Fig. 3.51). He exhibited crowding in his arches, maxillary canines developing high in the palate and with mesial eruption paths which appeared to endanger the integrity of the lateral incisor apices. The initial panoramic film exhibited both maxillary permanent canines with mesial eruption paths high in the palate and with a high probability of impaction

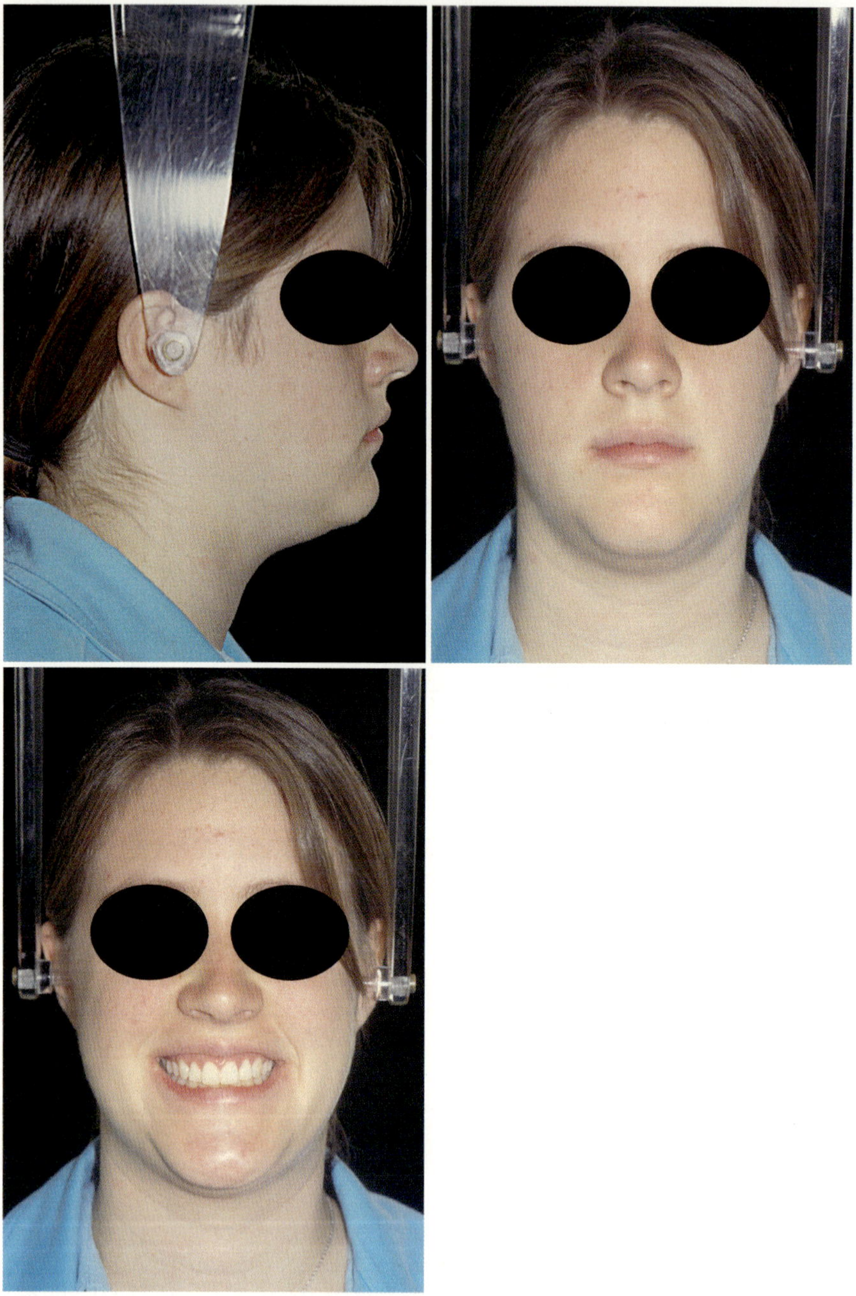

Figs. 3.43, 3.44, and 3.45 Six-year posttreatment facial views, age 17.6. Note good facial balance was maintained with no apparent skeletal or dental relapse. Patient continued using her retainers

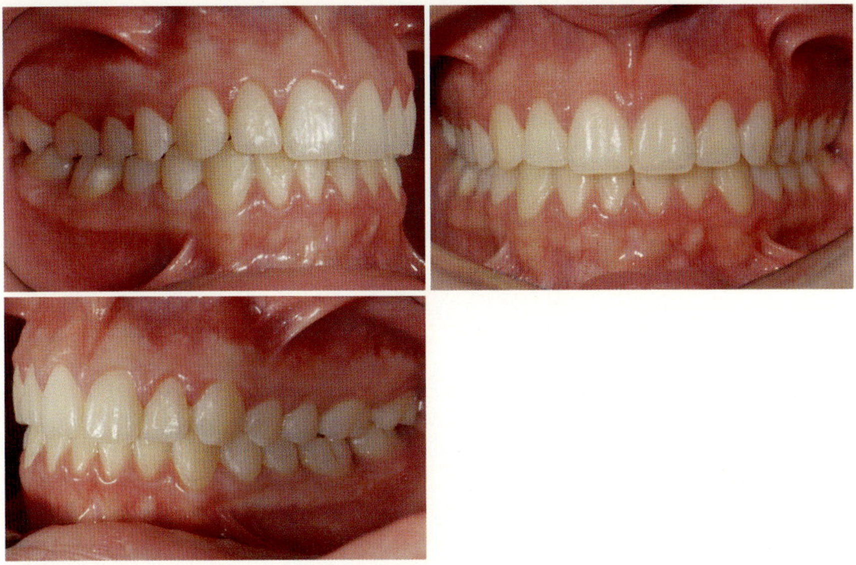

Figs. 3.46, 3.47, and 3.48 Six-year posttreatment intraoral views with teeth in occlusion. Note good stability with excellent occlusion and midline coincidence

Fig. 3.49 Six-year posttreatment cephalogram. ANB angle is now 2°. Good skeletal and dental relationships were maintained and there is lip competence. Note good occlusion. Third molars are still developing

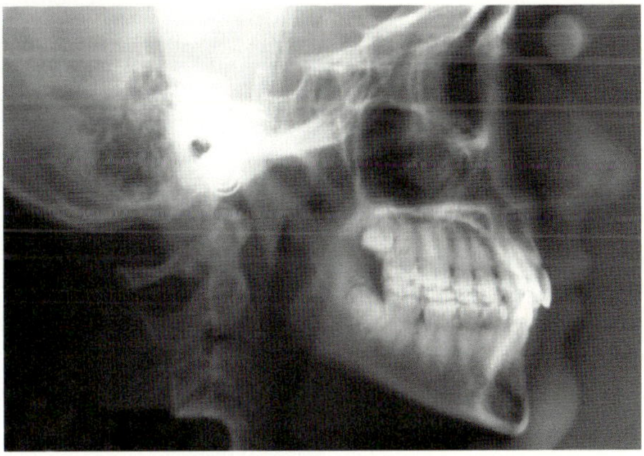

(Fig. 3.52). Due to his dental crowding, it was decided to institute a serial extraction therapy culminating with the extraction of two lower second bicuspids and two upper first bicuspids. The reason for extracting lower second bicuspids instead of lower first bicuspids was to protect his straight facial profile so it would not flatten.

Treatment began with the extraction of the four primary canines and the 4 first primary molars. Once the extraction areas had healed, a lower lingual holding arch was cemented on his permanent first molars and a maxillary removable plate was given. Four months later, his maxillary first bicuspids erupted and were extracted.

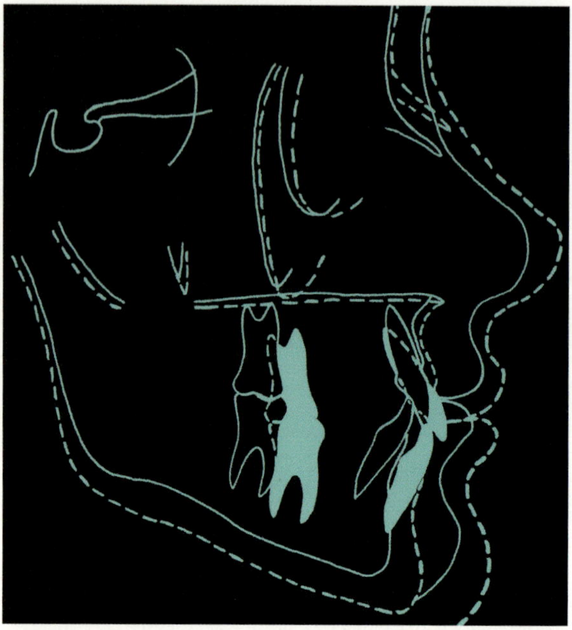

Fig. 3.50 Posttreatment cranial base superimposition of cephalogram tracings, ages 11.5 and 17.6. Note forward and downward mandibular growth while maxillary forward growth proceeded in the same direction but with less magnitude. Note good skeletal, dental, and facial relationships were maintained. Due to greater mandibular than maxillary growth, the chin is further forward

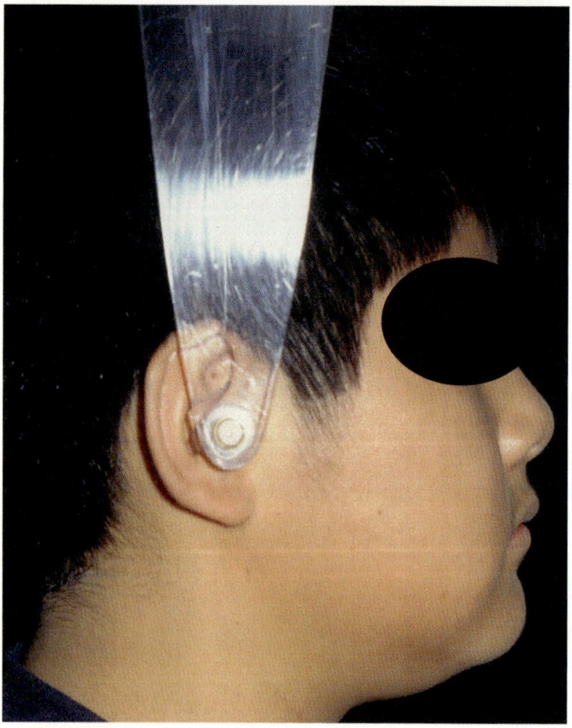

Fig. 3.51 Pretreatment facial profile view of a 9.11-year-old boy. Note straight profile

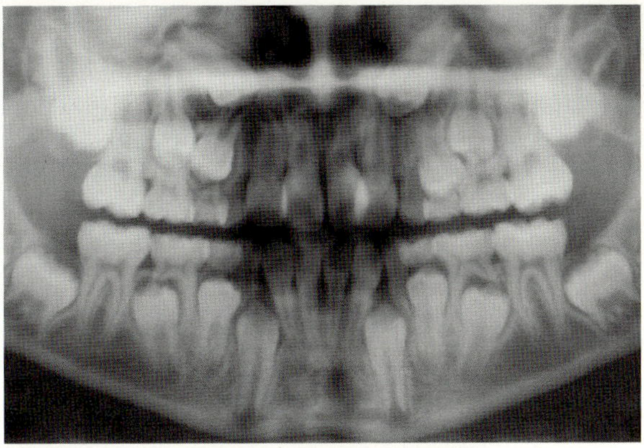

Fig. 3.52 Pretreatment panoramic radiograph. Note maxillary canines developing high in the plate and with mesial eruption paths, endangering the lateral incisor roots. Also note incisor crowding

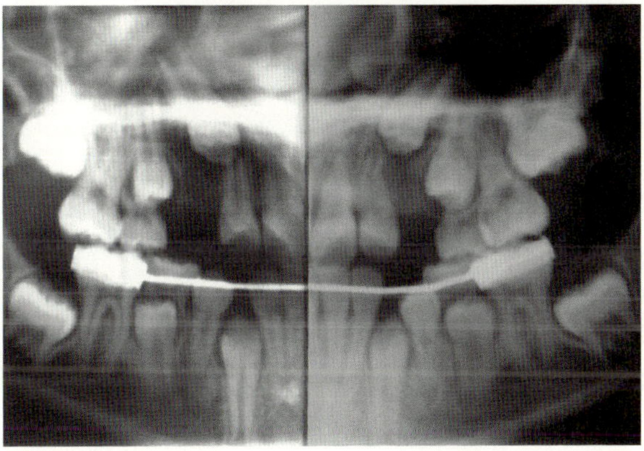

Fig. 3.53 Progress panoramic radiograph taken at age 10.5. Note that the maxillary canine eruption paths are still mesial; maxillary first bicuspids have already been extracted. Also note that a fixed lower holding lingual arch has been placed since maxillary and mandibular primary canines and primary first molars had been previously extracted. Not shown is a maxillary removable plate given to patient to prevent the maxillary incisors from spacing and to hold the extraction spaces open

Two months later, another panoramic film was taken to monitor the eruption path of the maxillary canines (Fig. 3.53). At this time, the second primary lower molars were extracted. Six months later, another panoramic film was taken to continue monitoring the eruption of the maxillary canines (Fig. 3.54). The lower second bicuspids had erupted sufficiently and were extracted. Six months later, an additional panoramic film was taken which revealed that the permanent canines were finally erupting in a normal path without endangering the integrity of the lateral incisor roots (Fig. 3.55). The canines had erupted sufficiently by age 14.0, so brackets were bonded to his teeth (Fig. 3.56) to close the remaining extraction spaces and to parallel the roots (Fig. 3.57). The posttreatment profile facial

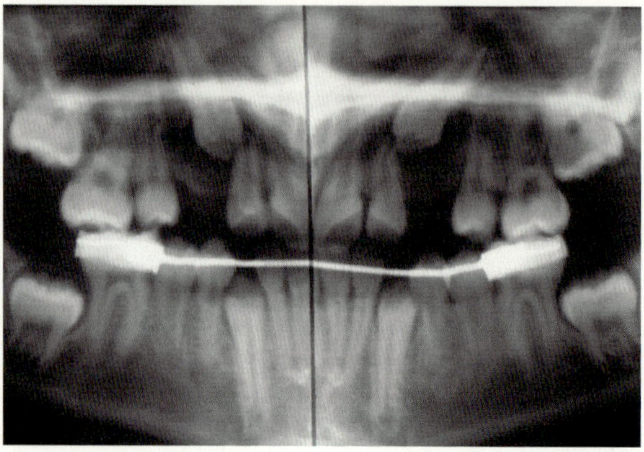

Fig. 3.54 Progress panoramic radiograph taken at age 10.11. Note that the maxillary canine eruption paths have improved and are now more vertical. Also note insufficient space for the eruption of the lower canines. Extraction of the lower second bicuspids was indicated to avoid flattening the patient's facial profile

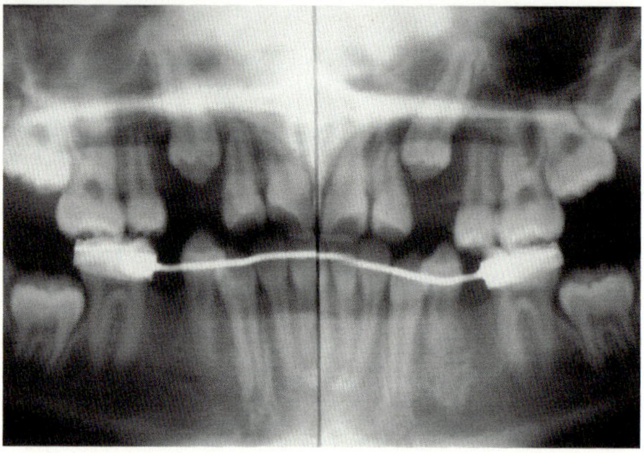

Fig. 3.55 Progress panoramic radiograph taken at age 11.5. Note that the maxillary canine eruption paths have improved even more and are now normal. Also note that the extraction of the lower second bicuspids has already been done. The lower first bicuspids are beginning to migrate distally giving space for the eruption of the lower canines

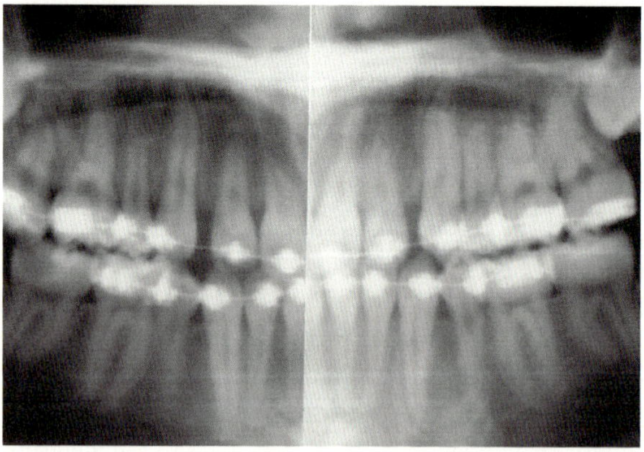

Fig. 3.56 Progress panoramic radiograph taken at age 14.0. Note that all canines have erupted and that full brackets have been bonded to close the remaining spaces and to parallel the roots

photograph taken at the age of 15.2 demonstrates that the flattening of his profile was indeed avoided (Fig. 3.58). This case illustrates the importance of seeing patients early enough to be able to change the eruption path of canines before they resorb incisor roots.

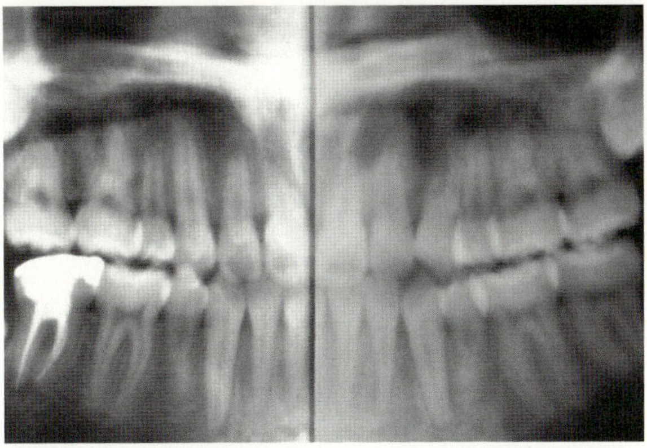

Fig. 3.57 Posttreatment panoramic radiograph taken at age 15.2. Note no EARR occurred. This case illustrates that the clinician can use this serial extraction method to change the mesial eruption paths of maxillary canines avoiding canine impactions and incisor root resorptions caused by these canines

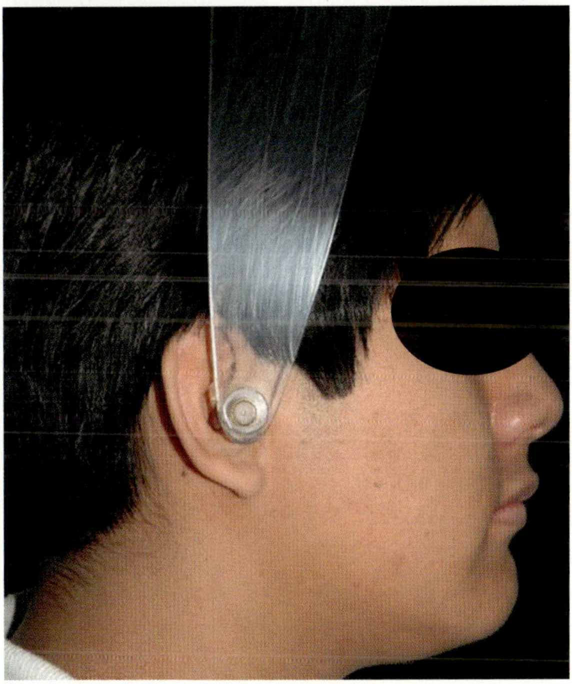

Fig. 3.58 Posttreatment facial profile view of a 15.2-year-old patient. Note maintenance of the straight profile in spite of four bicuspid extractions. The reason for the maintenance of his profile was that lower second bicuspids and upper first bicuspids were extracted (for a more detailed explanation, please review Chap. 2 of this book)

3.7.3 Serial Extraction to Modify Eruption Paths (Guidance of Eruption)

Serial extraction without fixed orthodontic appliances is also a root-sparing treatment regime. This alleviates dental crowding by guiding teeth to erupt closer to their ideal positions, thereby minimizing the need for extensive orthodontic tooth movements once all permanent teeth have erupted. Patients E and F, presented previously, are examples in which the extraction of primary teeth at an appropriate time (sometimes followed by premolar extractions) reduces the distance that an orthodontist has to move the teeth, thereby minimizing the risk of EARR development. Treatment time with fixed appliances is also reduced if teeth are guided to erupt closer to their final positions, which also minimizes the risk of EARR development.

3.7.4 Correction of Anterior Open Bite with a Palatal Tongue Spur Appliance

Anterior open bite has been associated with increased risk for EARR. This is thought to occur through jiggling forces from the tongue and lips [94]. Early interception of habits such as anterior tongue rest posture or digit sucking therefore minimizes the risk for EARR development as well and may be considered an orthodontic root-sparing treatment regime. The following case report of patient G is an example of how, by cementing a tongue spur reminding appliance, the anterior tongue rest posture can be modified. This in turn allows the incisors to erupt resulting in anterior open-bite closure, obviating the use of active orthodontic appliances.

Patient G was a 9-year-old healthy boy with a Class I anterior open-bite malocclusion. He exhibited a symmetric 6-mm dental open bite extending from lateral incisor to lateral incisor (Figs. 3.59 and 3.60). The crowns of the maxillary lateral incisors

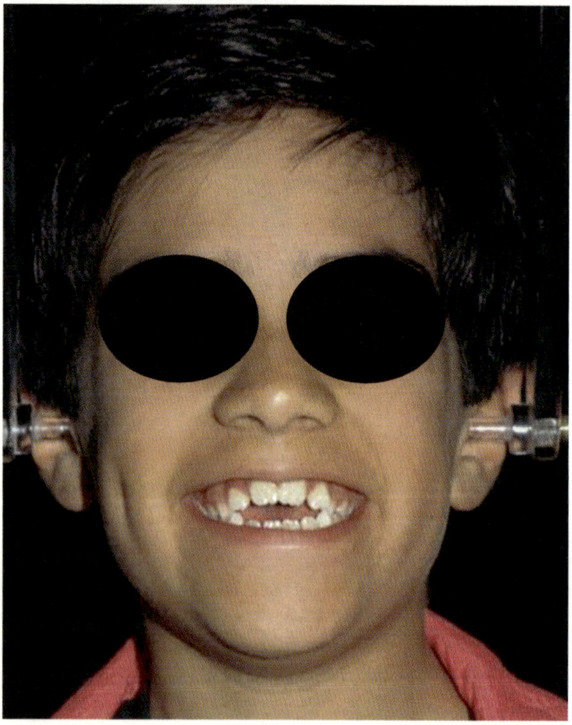

Fig. 3.59 Frontal facial view of a 9 year old boy with an anterior open bite

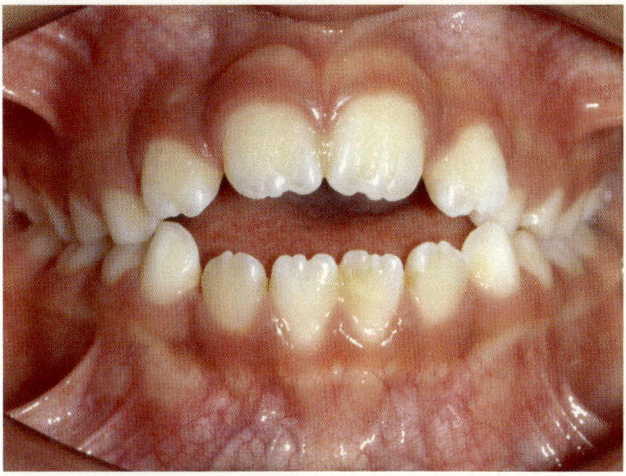

Fig. 3.60 Pretreatment intraoral photograph. Note anterior open bite, lingual crossbite of maxillary primary left canine, and distal inclination of the maxillary lateral incisor crowns

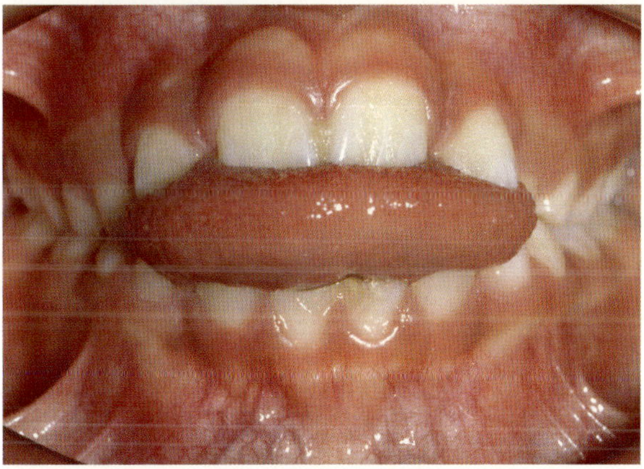

Fig. 3.61 Anterior tongue rest posture causing the open bite

had a distal inclination due to a mesial eruption path of the permanent canines against the roots of the lateral incisors. In addition, the maxillary left deciduous canine was in lingual crossbite (Fig. 3.60). An anterior tongue rest posture was noted (Fig. 3.61). There was no history of a digit-sucking habit and no respiration problems were noted. The patient also had normal skeletal cephalometric values and no family history of hyperdivergence. The patient and his parents were shown the abnormal anterior tongue resting posture of the patient. They were informed of the possibility that the open bite might not self-correct with orthodontic treatment due to the abnormal tongue rest posture. In the event the open bite did not self-correct, spur therapy was presented as an alternative. The treatment plan included extraction of deciduous maxillary canines (to help redirect the eruption path of the permanent canines), wearing of occipital pull headgear (to inhibit maxillary molar eruption and maxillary vertical posterior growth), and allowing the anterior open bite to self-correct. After 6 months of headgear treatment (Fig. 3.62), good rapport was established with the patient and his parents. Since the anterior open bite had not improved by this time

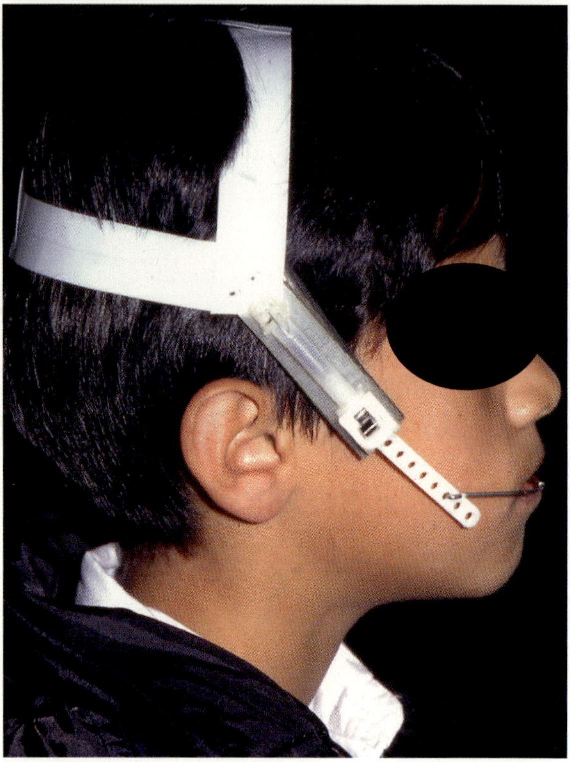

Fig. 3.62 Occipital traction facebow

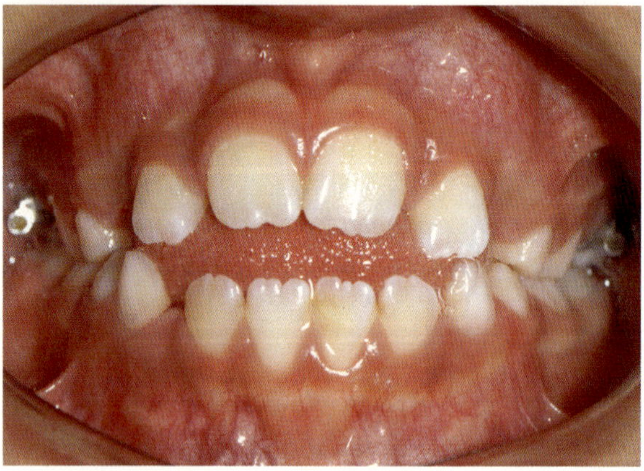

Fig. 3.63 Progress intraoral photograph 6 months into headgear treatment. There was no improvement in the anterior open bite

(Fig. 3.63), the patient and his parents consented to the spur method. A lingual arch with spurs (Figs. 3.64 and 3.65) was soldered to the maxillary first molar bands and cemented. The patient adapted well to the spurs (Fig. 3.66). The incisors erupted fully in the following 24 months, which closed the anterior open bite (Figs. 3.67,

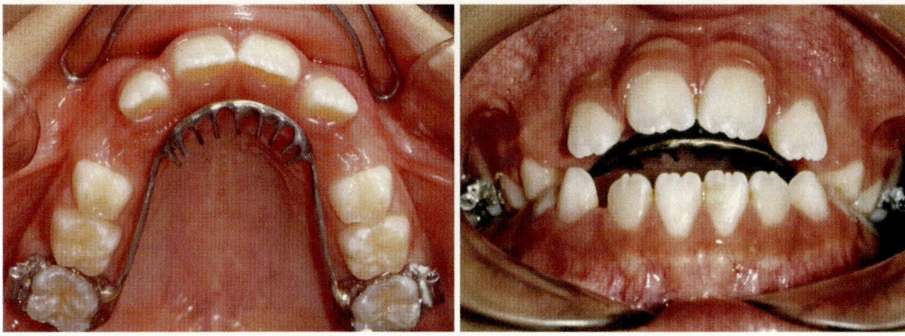

Figs. 3.64 and 3.65 Intraoral spur appliance

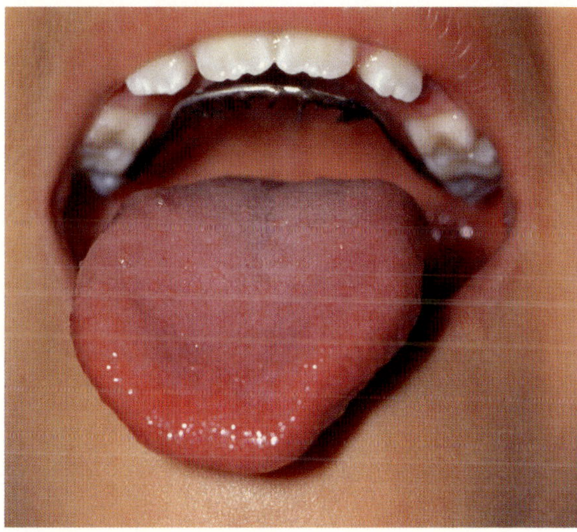

Fig. 3.66 Intraoral photograph of spurs and tongue taken 1 month after spur appliance cementation. There are no bruises on the tongue, which is probably due to a protective reflex

3.68, 3.69, and 3.70). In addition, the maxillary permanent canines were able to erupt uneventfully while the axial inclination of the lateral incisors self-corrected. Without treatment to resolve the patient's anterior open bite, if a self-correction had not occurred, many problems could have developed. These risks include an increased probability of incisor root resorption, molar wear due to the lack of a mutually protected occlusion, posterior crossbite due to a low tongue posture, or emotional consequences due to diminished dental esthetics during speech and smiling. In addition, the likelihood of a more complicated course of orthodontic treatment is greatly increased, possibly including a need for surgical correction. The lack of stability of corrected anterior open bite has been well documented. Huang et al. [119] and Justus [120] have demonstrated, however, long-term stability of anterior open-bite correction when *tongue spurs* are used to modify tongue posture.

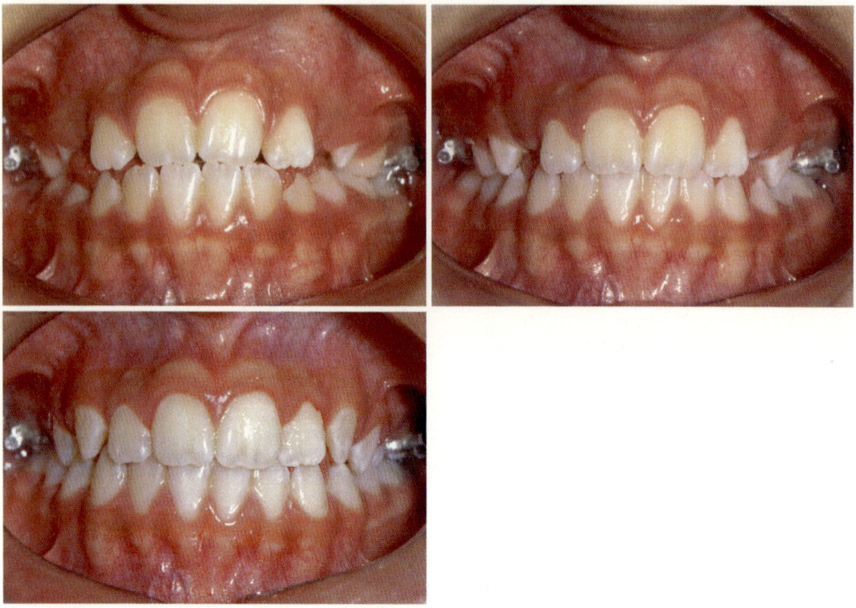

Figs. 3.67, 3.68, and 3.69 Progress intraoral photographs taken 12, 24, and 30 months after cementing the spur appliance. There has been full closure of the anterior open bite, probably due to the establishment of a new tongue rest posture encouraged by the spurs. No brackets were required

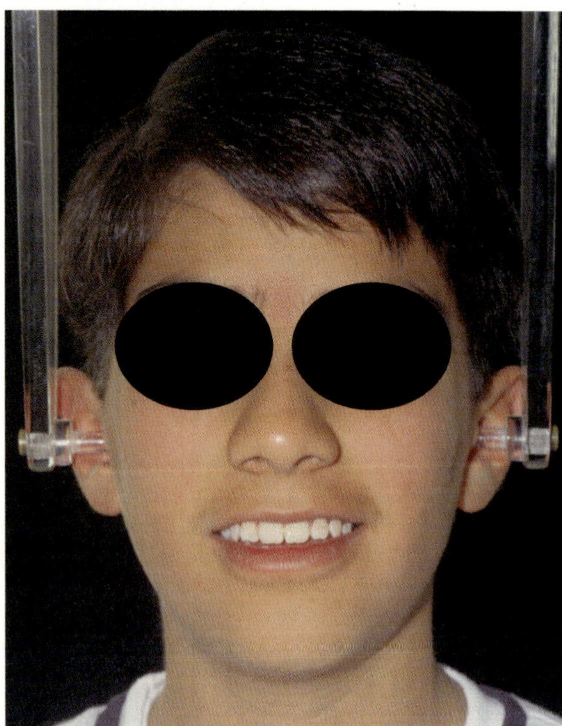

Fig. 3.70 Posttreatment frontal smiling photograph of the patient at 12 years of age

3.7.5 Orthognathic Surgery to Avoid Moving Teeth Large Distances and Against Cortical Plates

Orthognathic surgery can also be considered a root-sparing orthodontic treatment regime since the only orthodontic movements required are decompensatory. Unfortunately, the current trend is to avoid orthognathic surgery because insurance companies often refuse to pay for these operations. This trend puts patients at increased risk of EARR. Orthodontic treatment without orthognathic surgery in patients for whom surgery is indicated obligates the orthodontist to move teeth *large distances* which increases *treatment time*. Both factors, plus the *proximity of roots to cortical plates*, create a higher risk of EARR development. Patient A presented in Chap. 2 of this book serves as an example of the use of orthognathic surgery to avoid overcompensating tooth positions. The best EARR prevention measure in this circumstance is *not to treat* patients who require orthognathic surgery but who refuse to undergo the surgery.

3.8 Recommendations to Minimize or Avoid Malpractice Lawsuits

Elizabeth Franklin, the American Association of Orthodontists Insurance Company claims manager, in a personal communication, has shared that root resorption is one of several important causes of loss in orthodontic malpractice claims. Some root resorption claims, depending on the number of teeth involved and the degree of resorption, can result in significant claim settlements if the case is not defensible. Franklin has published extensively in the Risk Management Review Section of the AAO Bulletin giving specific examples of malpractice lawsuits [121, 122].

To minimize the risk for development of the severe form of EARR, as well as to reduce the chance for any subsequent lawsuit, orthodontic practice recommendations are the following:

- Obtain quality initial patient records, which include periapical radiographs of maxillary incisors.
- Obtain signed informed consent forms specifically outlining EARR.
- Look at siblings and parents' post-orthodontic periapical radiographs if available.
- Use treatment strategies that spare the root apices by minimizing the need for extensive tooth movements.
- Use light and well-distributed forces.
- Obtain periapical radiographs of maxillary incisors 6 months after fixed appliance placement *of every patient* to identify patients at risk.

If EARR is detected during orthodontic treatment:

- Inform the patient and/or parents.
- Change treatment plans if necessary.

- Interrupt treatment for approximately 3 months using passive arch wires.
- Reactivate arch wires every other month, alternating maxillary and mandibular adjustments.
- Avoid tooth movement against cortical plates.
- Obtain final patient records of excellent quality, which include periapical radiographs of maxillary incisors.

3.9 Concluding Remarks

Orthodontists are highly trained dental caregivers obligated to abide by the Hippocratic Oath of doing no harm. It is my hope that this third chapter will create awareness among clinicians that there are orthodontic and orthopedic treatment regimes designed precisely to minimize or even avoid the development of EARR. Successful treatment should begin at a young age so that the clinician can take advantage of *eruption guidance* and of *growth modification* when a Class II skeletal problem exists. Suggested treatment regimes outlined in this chapter minimize the distance that teeth need to be moved helping protect the patient from developing the severe form of EARR.

References

1. Fuss Z, Tsesis I, Lin S. Root resorption–diagnosis, classification and treatment choices based on stimulation factors. Dent Traumatol. 2003;19:175–82.
2. Proffit WR, Fields HW, Sarver DM. Contemporary orthodontic. 4th ed. Saint Louis: Mosby, Inc. USA; 2007. p. 279–83.
3. Weltman BJ. External root resorption and orthodontic treatment—assessment of the evidence. In: Huang GJ, Richmond S, Vig KWL, editors. Evidence-based orthodontics. Chichester: Wiley-Blackwell Publishing Ltd UK; 2011. p. 63–87.
4. Mirabella AD, Årtun J. Risk factors for apical root resorption of maxillary anterior teeth in adult orthodontic patients. Am J Orthod Dentofacial Orthop. 1995;108:48–55.
5. Lupi JE, Handelman CS, Sadowsky C. Prevalence and severity of apical root resorption and alveolar bone loss in orthodontically treated adults. Am J Orthod Dentofacial Orthop. 1996;109:28–37.
6. Taithongchai R, Sookkorn K, Killiany DM. Facial and dentoalveolar structure and the prediction of apical root shortening. Am J Orthod Dentofacial Orthop. 1996;110:296–302.
7. Sameshima GT, Sinclair PM. Predicting and preventing root resorption: part 1. Diagnostic factors. Am J Orthod Dentofacial Orthop. 2001;119:505–10.
8. Sameshima GT, Sinclair PM. Predicting and preventing root resorption: part II. Treatment factors. Am J Orthod Dentofacial Orthop. 2001;119:511–5.
9. Brin I, Tulloch JFC, Koroluk L, et al. External apical root resorption in Class II malocclusion: a retrospective review of 1-versus 2-phase treatment. Am J Orthod Dentofacial Orthop. 2003;124:151–6.
10. Remington DN, Joondeph DR, Årtun J, et al. Long-term evaluation of root resorption occurring during orthodontic treatment. Am J Orthod Dentofacial Orthop. 1989;96:43–6.

11. Kaley JD, Phillips C. Factors related to root resorption in edgewise practice. Angle Orthod. 1991;61:125–32.
12. Linge L, Linge BO. Patient characteristics and treatment variables associated with apical root resorption during orthodontic treatment. Am J Orthod Dentofacial Orthop. 1991;99:35–43.
13. Weltman B, Vig KWL, Fields HW, et al. Root resorption associated with orthodontic tooth movement: a systematic review. Am J Orthod Dentofacial Orthop. 2010;137:462–76.
14. Levander E, Malmgren O. Evaluation of the risk of root resorption during orthodontic treatment: a study of upper incisors. Eur J Orthod. 1988;10:30–8.
15. Otis L, Hong J, Tuncay O. Bone structure effect on root resorption. Orthod Craniofac Res. 2004;21:165–77.
16. Segal GR, Schiffman PH, Tuncay OH. Meta analysis of the treatment-related factors of external apical root resorption. Orthod Craniofac Res. 2004;7:71–8.
17. DeShields RW. A study of root resorption in treated Class II, Division I malocclusions. Angle Orthod. 1969;39:231–45.
18. Baumrind S, Korn EL, Boyd RL. Apical root resorption in orthodontically treated adults. Am J Orthod Dentofacial Orthop. 1996;110:311–20.
19. Casa MA, Faltin RM, Faltin K, et al. Root resorptions in upper first premolars after application of continuous torque moment. Intra-individual study. J Orofac Orthop. 2001;62:285–95.
20. Jimenez-Pellegrin C, Arana-Chavez VE. Root resorption in human mandibular first premolars after rotation as detected by scanning electron microscopy. Am J Orthod Dentofacial Orthop. 2004;126:178–84.
21. Fox N. Longer orthodontic treatment may result in greater external apical root resorption. Evid Based Dent. 2005;6:21.
22. McFadden WM, Engstrom C, Engstrom H, et al. A study of the relationship between incisor intrusion and root shortening. Am J Orthod Dentofacial Orthop. 1989;96:390–6
23. Sameshima GT, Sinclair PM. Characteristics of patients with severe root resorption. Orthod Craniofac Res. 2004;7:108–14.
24. Beck BW, Harris EF. Apical root resorption in orthodontically treated subjects: analysis of edgewise and light wire mechanics. Am J Orthod Dentofacial Orthop. 1994;105:350–61.
25. Dermaut LR, De Munck A. Apical root resorption of upper incisors caused by intrusive tooth movement: a radiographic study. Am J Orthod Dentofacial Orthop. 1986;90:321–6.
26. Harris DA, Jones AS, Darendeliler MA. Physical properties of root cementum: part 8. Volumetric analysis of root resorption craters after application of controlled intrusive light and heavy orthodontic forces: a microcomputed tomography scan study. Am J Orthod Dentofacial Orthop. 2006;130:639–47.
27. Barbagallo LJ, Jones AS, Petocz P, et al. Physical properties of root cementum: part 10. Comparison of the effects of invisible removable thermoplastic appliances with light and heavy orthodontic forces on premolar cementum. A microcomputed-tomography study. Am J Orthod Dentofacial Orthop. 2008;133:218–27.
28. Faltin RM, Faltin K, Sander FG, et al. Ultrastructure of cementum and periodontal ligament after continuous intrusion in humans: a transmission electron microscopy study. Eur J Orthod. 2001;23:35–49.
29. Chan EKM, Darendeliler MA. Exploring the third dimension in root resorption. Orthod Craniofac Res. 2004;7:64–70.
30. Chan E, Darendeliler MA. Physical properties of root cementum: part 5. Volumetric analysis of root resorption craters after application of light and heavy orthodontic forces. Am J Orthod Dentofacial Orthop. 2005;127:186–95.
31. Chan E, Darendeliler MA. Physical properties of root cementum: part 7. Extent of root resorption under areas of compression and tension. Am J Orthod Dentofacial Orthop. 2006;129:504–10.
32. Parker RJ, Harris EF. Directions of orthodontic tooth movements associated with external apical root resorption of the maxillary central incisor. Am J Orthod Dentofacial Orthop. 1998;114:672–83.

33. Han G, Huang S, Von den Hoff JW, et al. Root resorption after orthodontic intrusion and extrusion: an intraindividual study. Angle Orthod. 2005;75:912–8.
34. Costopoulos G, Nanda R. An evaluation of root resorption incident to orthodontic intrusion. Am J Orthod Dentofacial Orthop. 1996;109:543–8.
35. Thilander B, Rygh P, Reitan K. Tissue reactions in orthodontics. In: Graber TM, Vanarsdall RL, Vig KW, editors. Orthodontics: current principles and techniques. 4th ed. St Louis: C.V. Mosby; 2005.
36. Linge BO, Linge L. Apical root resorption in upper anterior teeth. Eur J Orthod. 1983;5:173–83.
37. Acar A, Canyurek U, Kocaaga M, et al. Continuous vs. discontinuous force application and root resorption. Angle Orthod. 1999;69:159–63.
38. Konoo T, Kim YJ, Gu GM, et al. Intermittent force in orthodontic tooth movement. J Dent Res. 2001;80:457–60.
39. Weiland F. Constant versus dissipating forces in orthodontics: the effect on initial tooth movement and root resorption. Eur J Orthod. 2003;25:335–42.
40. Owman-Moll P, Kurol J, Lundgren D. Continuous versus interrupted continuous orthodontic force related to early tooth movement and root resorption. Angle Orthod. 1995;65:395–401.
41. Brezniak N, Wasserstein A. Orthodontically induced inflammatory root resorption. Part II: the clinical aspects. Angle Orthod. 2002;72:180–4.
42. Brezniak N, Wasserstein A. Root resorption after orthodontic treatment: part 1. Literature review. Am J Orthod Dentofacial Orthop. 1993;103:62–6.
43. Ketcham AH. A preliminary report of an investigation of apical root resorption of vital permanent teeth. Int J Orthod. 1927;13:97–127.
44. Pandis N, Nasika M, Polychronopoulou A, et al. External apical root resorption in patients treated with conventional and self-ligating brackets. Am J Orthod Dentofacial Orthop. 2008;134:646–51.
45. Blake M, Woodside DG, Pharoah MJ. A radiographic comparison of apical root resorption after orthodontic treatment with the edgewise and speed appliances. Am J Orthod Dentofacial Orthop. 1995;108:76–84.
46. Janson GR, De Luca Canto G, Martins DR, et al. A radiographic comparison of apical root resorption after orthodontic treatment with 3 different fixed appliance techniques. Am J Orthod Dentofacial Orthop. 1999;118:262–73.
47. Malmgren O, Goldson L, Hill C, et al. Root resorption after orthodontic treatment of traumatized teeth. Am J Orthod. 1982;82:487–91.
48. Goldson L, Henrikson CO. Root resorption during Begg treatment: a longitudinal roentgenologic study. Am J Orthod. 1975;68:55–66.
49. TenHoeve A, Mulie RM. The effects of antero-postero incisor repositioning on the palatal cortex as studied with laminagraphy. J Clin Orthod. 1976;10:804–22.
50. McNab S, Battistutta D, Taverne A, et al. External apical root resorption following orthodontic treatment. Angle Orthod. 2000;70:227–32.
51. Lew K. Intrusion and apical resorption of mandibular incisors in Begg treatment: anchorage bend or curve? Aust Orthod J. 1990;11:164–8.
52. Alexander SA. Levels of root resorption associated with continuous arch and sectional arch mechanics. Am J Orthod Dentofacial Orthop. 1996;110:321–4.
53. Scott P, DiBiase AT, Sherriff M, et al. Alignment efficiency of Damon3 self-ligating and conventional orthodontic bracket systems: a randomized clinical trial. Am J Orthod Dentofacial Orthop. 2008;134:470.e1–8.
54. Hartsfield Jr JK, Everett ET, Al-Qawasmi RA. Genetic factors in external apical root resorption and orthodontic treatment. Crit Rev Oral Biol Med. 2004;15:115–22.
55. Hamilton RS, Gutmann JL. Endodontic-orthodontic relationships: a review of integrated treatment planning challenges. Int Endod J. 1999;32:343–60.
56. Drysdale C, Gibbs SL, Ford TR. Orthodontic management of root-filled teeth. Br J Orthod. 1996;23:255 60.

57. Newman WG. Possible etiologic factors in external root resorption. Am J Orthod. 1975;67:522–39.
58. McNab S, Battistutta D, Taverne A, et al. External apical root resorption of posterior teeth in asthmatics after orthodontic treatment. Am J Orthod Dentofacial Orthop. 1999;116:545–51.
59. Kjaer I. Morphological characteristics of dentitions developing excessive root resorption during orthodontic treatment. Eur J Orthod. 1995;17:25–34.
60. Smale I, Årtun J, Behbehani F, et al. Apical root resorption 6 months after initiation of fixed orthodontic appliance therapy. Am J Orthod Dentofacial Orthop. 2005;128:57–67.
61. Thongudomporn U, Freer TJ. Anomalous dental morphology and root resorption during orthodontic treatment: a pilot study. Aust Orthod J. 1998;15:162–7.
62. Lee RY, Årtun J, Alonzo TA. Are dental anomalies risk factors for apical root resorption in orthodontic patients? Am J Orthod Dentofacial Orthop. 1999;116:187–95.
63. English H. External apical root resorption as a consequence of orthodontic treatment. J N Z Soc Periodontol. 2001;86:17–23.
64. Al-Qawasmi RA, Hartsfield Jr JK, Everett ET, et al. Genetic predisposition to external apical root resorption. Am J Orthod Dentofacial Orthop. 2003;123:242–52.
65. Harris EF, Kineret SE, Tolley EA. A heritable component for external apical root resorption in patients treated orthodontically. Am J Orthod Dentofacial Orthop. 1997;111:301–9.
66. Ngan DCS, Kharbanda OP, Byloff FK, et al. The genetic contribution to orthodontic root resorption: a retrospective twin study. Aust Orthod J. 2004;20:1–9.
67. Al-Qawasmi RA, Hartsfield Jr JK, Everett ET, et al. Genetic predisposition to external apical root resorption in orthodontic patients: linkage of chromosome-18 marker. J Dent Res. 2003;82:356–60.
68. Bollen AM. Large overjet and longer teeth are associated with more root resorption when treated orthodontically. J Evid Based Dent Pract. 2002;2:44–5
69. Igarashi K, Adachi H, Mitani H, et al. Inhibitory effect of topical administration of a bisphosphonate (risedronate) on root resorption incident to orthodontic tooth movement in rats. J Dent Res. 1996;75:1644–9.
70. Adachi H, Igarashi K, Mitani H, et al. Effects of topical administration of a bisphosphonate (risedronate) on orthodontic tooth movement in rats. J Dent Res. 1994;73:1478–86.
71. Attati I, Hammarstrom L. Root surface defects in rat molar induced by 1-hydroxyethylidene-1, 1-bisphosphonate. Acta Odontol Scand. 1996;54:59–65.
72. Attati I, Hellsing E, Hammarstrom L. Orthodontically induced root resorption in rat molars after 1-hydroxyethylidene-1, 1-bisphosphonate injection. Acta Odontol Scand. 1996;54:102–8.
73. Villa PA, Oberti G, Moncada CA, et al. Pulp-dentine complex changes and root resorption during intrusive orthodontic tooth movement in patients prescribed nabumetone. J Endod. 2005;31:61–6.
74. Poumpros E, Loberg E, Engstrom C. Thyroid function and root resorption. Angle Orthod. 1994;64:389–93.
75. Shirazi M, Dehpour AR, Jefari F. The effect of thyroid hormone on orthodontic tooth movement in rats. J Clin Pediatr Dent. 1999;23:259–64.
76. Loberg EL, Engstrom C. Thyroid administration to reduce root resorption. Angle Orthod. 1994;64:395–9.
77. Christiansen RL. Commentary: thyroxine administration and its effects on root resorption. Angle Orthod. 1994;64:399–400.
78. Horiuchi A, Hotokezaka H, Kobayashi K. Correlation between cortical plate proximity and apical root resorption. Am J Orthod Dentofacial Orthop. 1998;114:311–8.
79. Rygh P, Reitan K. Ultrastructural changes in the periodontal ligament incident to orthodontic tooth movement. Trans Eur Orthod Soc. 1972;393–405.
80. Goldie RS, King GJ. Root resorption and tooth movement in orthodontically treated, calcium-deficient, and lactating rats. Am J Orthod. 1984;85:424–30.
81. Midgett RJ, Shaye R, Fruge Jr JF. The effect of altered bone metabolism on orthodontic tooth movement. Am J Orthod. 1981;80:256–62.

82. Davidovitch Z, Godwin SL, Park YG, et al. The etiology of root resorption. In: McNamara JA, Trotman CA, editors. Orthodontic treatment: the management of unfavorable sequelae. Ann Arbor: University of Michigan Press; 1996. p. 93–117.
83. Andreasen JO. External root resorption: its implication in dental traumatology, paedodontics, periodontics, orthodontics and endodontics. Int Endod J. 1985;18:109–18.
84. Mandall N, Lowe C, Worthington H, et al. Which orthodontic archwire sequence? A randomized clinical trial. Eur J Orthod. 2006;28:561–6.
85. Brezniak N, Wasserstein A. Orthodontically induced inflammatory root resorption. Part 1: the basic science aspects. Angle Orthod. 2002;72:175–9.
86. Wickwire NA, McNeil MH, Norton LA, et al. The effects of tooth movement upon endodontically treated teeth. Angle Orthod. 1974;44:235–42.
87. Taner T, Ciger S, Sencift Y. Evaluation of apical root resorption following extraction therapy in subjects with class I and class II malocclusions. Eur J Orthod. 1999;21:491–6.
88. Harris EF, Robinson QC, Woods MA. An analysis of causes of apical root resorption in patients not treated orthodontically. Quintessence Int. 1993;24:417–28.
89. Mavragani M, Boe OE, Wisth PJ, et al. Changes in root length during orthodontic treatment: advantages for immature teeth. Eur J Orthod. 2002;24:91–7.
90. Reitan K. Initial tissue behaviour during apical root resorption. Angle Orthod. 1974;44:68–82.
91. Harris EF, Baker WC. Loss of root length and crestal bone height before and during treatment in adolescent and adult orthodontic patients. Am J Orthod Dentofacial Orthop. 1990;98:463–9.
92. Bishara SE, von Wald L, Jakobsen JR. Changes in root length from early to mid-adulthood: resorption or apposition? Am J Orthod Dentofacial Orthop. 1999;115:563–8.
93. Spurrier SW, Hall SH, Joondeph DR, et al. A comparison of apical root resorption during orthodontic treatment in endodontically treated and vital teeth. Am J Orthod Dentofacial Orthop. 1990;97:130–4.
94. Harris EF, Butler ML. Patterns of incisor root resorption before and after orthodontic correction of cases with anterior open bite. Am J Orthod Dentofacial Orthop. 1992;101:112–9.
95. Vlaskalic V, Boyd RL, Baumrind S. Etiology and sequelae of root resorption. Semin Orthod. 1998;4:124–31.
96. Årtun J, Smale I, Behbehani F, et al. Apical root resorption six and 12 months after initiation of fixed orthodontic appliance therapy. Angle Orthod. 2005;75:919–26.
97. Levander E, Malmgren O, Eliasson S. Evaluation of root resorption in relation to two orthodontic treatment regimes. A clinical experimental study. Eur J Orthod. 1994;16:223–8.
98. Kalkwarf KL, Krejci RF, Pao YC. Effect of apical root resorption on periodontal support. J Prosthet Dent. 1986;56:317–9.
99. Cureton SL, Regennitter FJ, Yancey JM. Clinical vs. quantitative assessment of headgear compliance. Am J Orthod Dentofacial Orthop. 1993;104:277–84.
100. Nguyen QV, Bezemer PD, Habets SL, et al. A systematic review of the relationship between overjet size and traumatic dental injuries. Eur J Orthod. 1999;21:503–15.
101. Koroluk L, Tulloch JFC, Phillips C. Incisor trauma and early treatment for Class II, Division 1 malocclusion. Am J Orthod Dentofacial Orthop. 2003;123:117–26.
102. Årtun J, Behbehani F, Al-Jame B, et al. Incisor trauma in an adolescent Arab population: prevalence, severity and occlusal risk factors. Am J Orthod Dentofacial Orthop. 2005;128:347–52.
103. Kaste LM, Gift HC, Bhat M, et al. Prevalence of incisor trauma in persons 6 to 50 years of age: United States, 1988–1991. J Dent Res. 1996;75(Spec iss):696–705.
104. Justus R. Letters to the Editor. Are there any advantages of early Class II treatment? Am J Orthod Dentofacial Orthop. 2008;134:717–8.
105. Huang G, English J, Ferguson D, et al. Functional appliances and long-term effects on mandibular growth. Am J Orthod Dentofacial Orthop (Readers' Forum). 2005;128:271–2.

106. O'Brien K, Wright J, Conboy F, et al. Effectiveness of early orthodontic treatment with the twin-block appliance: a multicenter randomized controlled trial. Part 1: dental and skeletal effects. Am J Orthod Dentofacial Orthop. 2003;124:234–43.
107. Tulloch JFC, Proffit WR, Phillips C. Outcomes in a 2-phase randomized clinical trial of early Class II treatment. Am J Orthod Dentofacial Orthop. 2004;125:657–67.
108. Moore AW. Orthodontic treatment factors in Class II malocclusion. Am J Orthod Dentofacial Orthop. 1959;45:323–52.
109. Wieslander L. The effects of orthodontic treatment on the concurrent development of the craniofacial complex. Am J Orthod Dentofacial Orthop. 1963;49:15–27.
110. Jakobsson SO. Cephalometric evaluation of treatment effect on Class II, Division 1 malocclusions. Am J Orthod Dentofacial Orthop. 1967;53:446–57.
111. Wieslander L. The effect of force on craniofacial development. Am J Orthod Dentofacial Orthop. 1974;65:531–8.
112. Melsen B. Effects of cervical anchorage during and after treatment: an implant study. Am J Orthod Dentofacial Orthop. 1978;73:526–40.
113. Baumrind S, Molthen R, West EE, et al. Distal displacement of the maxilla and the upper first molar. Am J Orthod Dentofacial Orthop. 1979;75:630–40.
114. Derringer K. A cephalometric study to compare the effects of cervical traction and Andresen therapy in the treatment of Class II, Division 1 malocclusion: part 1-skeletal changes. Br J Orthod. 1990;17:33–46.
115. Justus R. Finalización en Ortodoncia. In: Interlandi S, editor. Ortodoncia–Bases para la Iniciación. Sao Paulo: Editorial Artes Médicas; 2002. p. 533–46.
116. Fidler BC, Artun J, Joondeph DR, et al. Long-term stability of Class II malocclusions with successful occlusal results at end of active treatment. Am J Orthod Dentofacial Orthop. 1995;107:276–85.
117. Ericson S, Kurol J. Early treatment of palatally erupting maxillary canines by extraction of the primary canines. Eur J Orthod. 1988;10:283–95.
118. Bonetti GA, Zanarini M, Parenti SI, et al. Extraction of deciduous canines and first molars to prevent ectopic eruption of permanent canines. Am J Orthod Dentofacial Orthop. 2011;139:316–23.
119. Huang GJ, Justus R, Kennedy DB, et al. Stability of anterior open bite treated with crib therapy. Angle Orthod. 1990;60:17–26.
120. Justus R. Correction of anterior open bite with spurs: long-term stability. World J Orthod. 2001;2:219–31.
121. Franklin E. Losing sleep over malpractice claims. AAO Bulletin. Risk Management Review. Saint Louis, Missouri, USA. Jan/Feb 2005.
122. Franklin E. Prolonged orthodontic treatment increases exposure to malpractice claims: take steps to reduce risk. AAO Bulletin. Risk Management Review. Saint Louis, Missouri, USA Apr/May 2005.

Index

R. Justus, *Iatrogenic Effects of Orthodontic Treatment: Decision-Making in Prevention, Diagnosis, and Treatment*, DOI 10.1007/978-3-319-18353-4